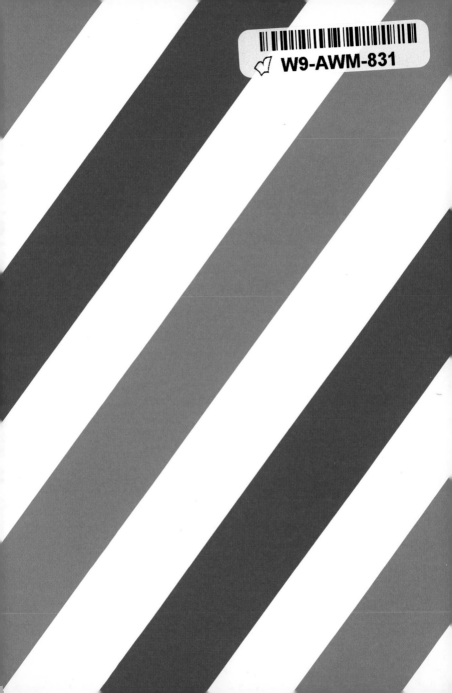

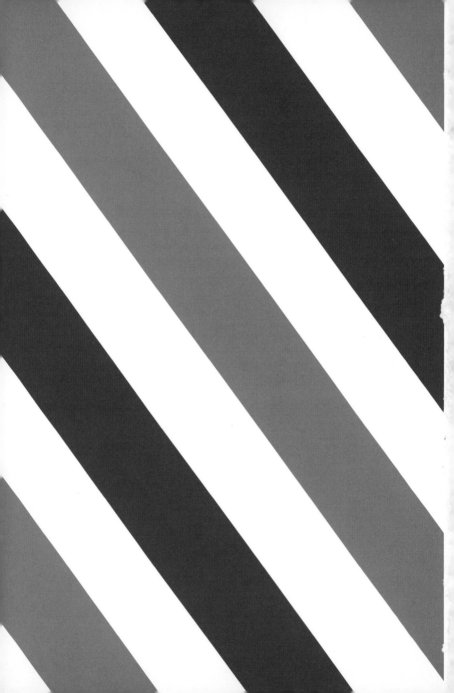

The
BARBER
Book

The BARBER Book

Edited by Giulia Pivetta
Illustrations by
Matteo Guarnaccia

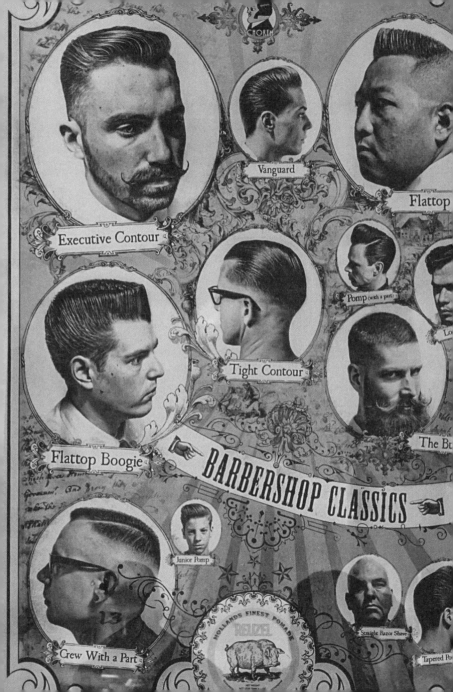

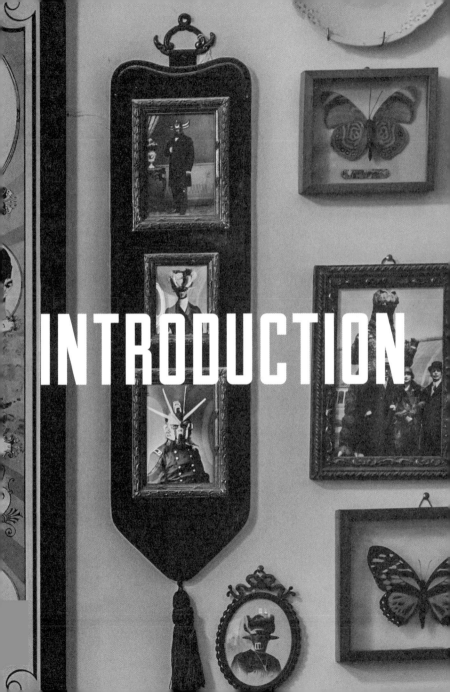

INTRODUCTION

Long or short, pomaded or natural, even left bald —
hair is a crucial social and cultural indicator, an
instant visual cue of role and gender. More intimate,
more personal, than clothing, it is a part of the body
that can be modified. It reminds us of the most
fundamental part of our being, a record of our origins
as a species, our animal nature. To style it is to
tame it; to reveal (or hide) a person's background
and even his or her philosophy. Hair is a form of
cultural shorthand, which, once deciphered, can spell
out entire sentences and stories. Hair expresses
personality in a direct way; it is a mirror that reflects
individual, collective and stylistic histories.

Every culture around the world has an established
set of symbolic values regarding hair. Some even
consider hair the source of man's vital force and
a point of direct connection with divinity. Male facial
hair is a secondary sexual characteristic, like breasts
on women. To touch someone's hair is an act of great
intimacy. Men of the third millennium worldwide
share a need for their hair to be loved and cared for.
This is where the barber steps in. His mastery of hair,
including moustaches and beards, has given rise
to a unique space — the barber shop — where rituals
of male bonding and grooming can blossom.

Among our ways of physically communicating
who we are, hair is the one that can be most readily
modified, the one that best suits a sudden change.
If we don't like the style, it doesn't matter: we know

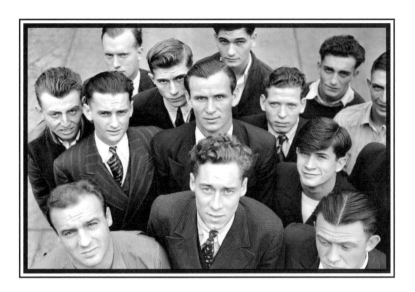

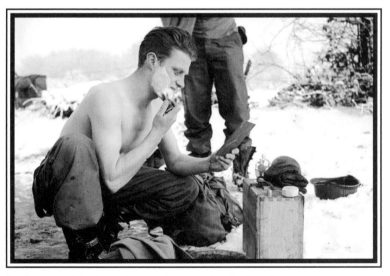

Top: Recruits waiting for medical examination and outfits, Fort Slocum NY, 1940
Bottom: US soldier shaving during the Battle of the Bulge, Belgium, 1945

it will grow back. We can manipulate its shape, its colour and its length quite easily, and a simple change in volume can give one the appearance of a new face and a new personality. Societies past and present have controlled and regulated hairstyles, first by tradition and religion and later through fashion. Hairstyles have not only been used to define roles, but also to clearly mark a difference between the sexes.

By the point at which we start this book, the middle years of the twentieth century, men in the West had for decades kept hair short or hidden under a hat, while the norm for women was to have long hair, often tied back. The concept of masculinity was tightly connected to the idea of the patriarch, the warrior, the head of the family — a model that endured into the early 1940s. World War II shook } up more than just the political landscape. Its after-effects included a total rethink of personal appearance, including hair. As the economy began to boom, a swelling generation of young people — teenagers — sparked social revolution. The male archetype of old was challenged: rock 'n' roll was born. By the 1970s attitudes to hair at their extreme were polarized between the Hippies, who never cut it, and the Skinheads, who kept only millimetres. The study of the intervening years, through men's hairstyles, gives us an understanding of how these changes came about. We will consider various types of cut — from controlled and elegant, to rebellious —

including some that defy categorization, such as the crazy haircuts worn by artists, on whom society has usually thought it better to suspend judgement. Each of these styles is the statement of a particular personality, sometimes of an ideology. This book is not a global survey but focuses on social cultures and subcultures of Britain, Europe and the United States during a period of change whose effects — and styles — still resonate today.

THE WAR YEARS AND BEYOND: HAIRCUTS OF CONTROL

Men stepped smartly into the 1940s wearing a uniform. Britain and much of Europe had been at war since 1939, and by 1941 the British Commonwealth (including Australia, New Zealand, Canada and South Africa), the Soviet Union, Japan and the US had joined them. What stayed under control, largely, was hair. Concepts such as enhanced masculinity, national belonging and cohesion, whether imposed or not, characterize the World War II period. For those living on the front lines, between barracks and battlefields, discipline and hygiene standards imposed short hair or hair kept in place with plenty of brilliantine.

As primary channels for the homogenization process, the armed forces have always played a central role in the control and regulation of society, as school does during childhood. Historically, these two strongly hierarchical institutions blended individuals into uniformed groups in order to attenuate any individualism and personal characteristics. One way to achieve this was through imposing a regulation haircut. Every national army had a specific haircut, derived from military traditions or influenced by a more modern concept of elegance. This explains how hairstyles have emerged as signs of national identity in the past: the Crew Cut and the Ivy League are emblematic of the United States; the Undercut, before its rediscovery by David Bowie, was once specifically German. More than that, some haircuts came to imply membership of a particular unit: a longer-length, Brylcreemed Executive Contour was the glamorous style of the RAF pilot.

Civilian populations adopted these controlled, structured haircuts, partly to emulate their heroes, partly to fit in and partly because they were easy. Easy to shape and easy to maintain, they required little personal involvement in styling. Important exceptions were the youth subcultures connected to jazz music, such as the Zoot Suiters in the United States, the Swing Kids in Germany, the Zazous in France and the Gagà in Italy: haircuts of rebellion. Fashions carried by the rhythm of swing music even made their way to the front, hidden under helmets but ready to be revealed to impress girls when off duty. Frequently, these infringements of military rules would be severely and publicly punished in the

name of upholding morality and respect. When
the Screaming Eagles parachute regiment dropped
into Normandy wearing Mohawks, it was the haircut's
links to an ancient warrior nation of the Iroquois
League that saved them from disgrace: rebellious,
but fitting.

The Slick Back was a controlled haircut that used
pomade to disguise its rakish lengths. It enjoyed
popularity from the turn of the twentieth century, but
it was Rudolph Valentino who inspired a generation
of men to seduce with a hairstyle, his shiny mane
the epitome of devilish good looks and *savoir-faire*.
In the 1930s and early 1940s men such as Humphrey
Bogart oozed Slick Back charm, the natural
descendants of the ultimate *tombeur de femmes*.
The look enjoyed a resurgence at the end of the war,
when the dominance of military cuts slowly receded.

The process of style liberation began with
minority groups aware of the fact that even the
slightest variation to the standard rule would give
them visibility. Stepping away from the mainstream
in order to follow their fashion creed, these brave men
sometimes jeopardized their own safety and
reputation in the process. Every extra inch of hair,
every curl out of place, every additional care given
to hair became a matter of public concern. In 1943
the Zoot Suiters of Los Angeles, who liked their
trousers wide and their jackets to the knee, faced
running battles with servicemen in the streets.

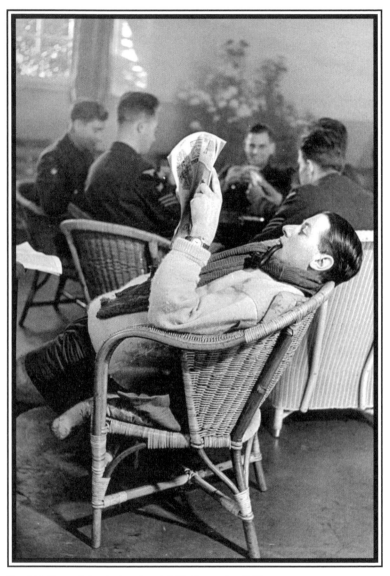

Royal Air Force pilots relaxing at a rehabilitation centre, 1942

After the war, Europe witnessed a softening of the sartorial rules as the long period of reconstruction began and citizens tried to leave the horrors of the past few years behind. Things were different in the United States, where a nation buoyed by victory (and with much of its infrastructure intact) received a new masculine typology, a vision of man who embodied the optimism of the American Way of Life. He had a singular mission: to spread freedom, equality and the need for consumer goods. Dreamt up by the admen of Madison Avenue in the 1950s, his short, neat hair was emblematic of his strict moral code and dedication to hard work. President Eisenhower (1953–61), who had served as a general, was the perfect representative of this style and pugnacious world view, in which the continuity with military tradition was visible and accepted outside the barracks. The military Crew Cut crossed over into schools and everyday life, and lasted until the early 1960s, standing as a symbol of order, cleanliness, good manners, good physical condition and adhesion to the social system.

THE 1950S: THE ECONOMIC BOOM AND THE BIRTH OF ROCK 'N' ROLL

During the Cold War, the United States and the Soviet Union faced each other not only on the political battlefield, but also in a cultural struggle. Respectively, they represented the individualistic world of consumerism and economic success, and the world of collective solidarity and shared social achievements: capitalism versus communism. These two superpowers also created new male archetypes, one defined by the Madison Avenue advertising agencies and one defined by party officials. Josef Stalin (who died in 1953) wore an iconic moustache that invited imitation; the Russian people were encouraged not to follow fashion but to look for enduring styles.

Communism outside the USSR found photogenic heroes in the Cuban Revolution, which came with its own identifiable hairstyle. The *Barbudos* grew their beards as a matter of pride and dedication, vowing only to trim them in the event of victory. Growing an Untamed Beard, or going 'full beard', appealed to young people in the West who idolized Fidel Castro and Che Guevara as freedom fighters and admired their outward commitment to a cause.

The American Dream was a rather sterile vision of life, rejecting natural sensuality: physicality was channelled towards sports. The very short hair worn by the military, elite school students and businessmen expressed an ongoing desire to exercise control. (The reality of suburban life has been explored in film and literature to an extent that the 1950s' dream of Doris Day and Rock Hudson has been all but supplanted by images of a seething underbelly of repression, as seen in David Lynch's 1986 film *Blue Velvet*.) Alternatives to the Madison

Avenue cut were offered by the Caesar and the Italiano styles.

Hollywood decamped to Rome during the 1950s, to the Cinecittà studios, and Italian modernism reigned in design and style. 'Sword and sandal' epics such as *Julius Caesar* (1953) offered a haircut that flattered a man with imperial ambitions, though it never really took off beyond the acting fraternity. The Italiano promised a life of sunshine and espressos. Outside Italy it found traction in Britain, where it was customized by the teenage Mods, who wore Italian suits and rode around on Vespas.

The threat to the clean-cut, all-American, mom's-apple-pie man, when it came, came not from the USSR or Cuba, but from within US society itself. A new mania — rock 'n' roll — emerged out of the African American and Latino communities. The passion for hair pomades among these populations made them subject to the mockery of white public opinion, which labelled them 'greasy': the hairstyles were well groomed and shiny, coated in brilliantine. But the music, rooted in bebop jazz, and the style, spoke to a new breed of young white adult. Among the first to spot the appeal were the prototype Hipsters of the Beat Generation, Jack Kerouac and Allen Ginsberg, who inspired a legacy of anti-mainstream couch-surfers that survives to this day.

The real revolution of the Fifties economic boom was the birth of a new figure — the teenager. Madison

Avenue conceived teenagers as consumers, pampering and spoiling them with exclusive products, but this newborn creature unexpectedly dodged any kind of control and social programme. Young people no longer aspired to become adults, but instead were determined to enjoy their adolescence in itself, claim their own identity and freedoms and make them last as long as possible. Rock 'n' roll became the key element of expression in this intergenerational gap, offering an ideal backdrop to youthful exuberance and adventure.

Teenagers found their idol in Elvis Presley, whose voice erupted onto the airwaves in 1954. His bass-baritone took black music to the top of the white hit parade, while his good looks, physicality and well-groomed quiff dominated cinema and television screens. Presley was a new kind of man, a man who, despite the predominant puritanical moral code, did not hide his narcissism or his sex appeal. The adult world was rattled: in its eyes this craze was connected to myths and distractions from the lower social classes. For the average middle-aged male, rock 'n' roll and delinquency were inextricably linked. The greasy quiff was their emblem.

During the 1950s subcultures proliferated in the United States at an enormous rate. Bikers, surfers, hot rodders, beatniks — all offered new ways of escape. The US no longer yielded the reassuring face of John Wayne or Harry Mancini's cocktail music, but Marlon Brando's sneer and Jerry Lee Lewis's fiery rhythms. These enticing models were seized upon by the youth of the Western world. In Britain, the Teddy Boys created their own mix, adding the recognizable quiff to customized suits in Edwardian style. Italian American youth gangs of New York and the Rockabillies of the Deep South exaggerated rock 'n' roll style, blended it with country music, and provided a new aesthetic and existential model for young rebels. Hollywood amplified and relaunched its essential character in personalities portrayed by actors such as Tony Curtis, Dean Martin and James Dean. Think *Rebel Without a Cause* (1955). Backcombed and brilliantine hairstyles came to stand for nonconformity, diversity and subversion. Mavericks and marginalized groups wore a style defying core aesthetic standards to express their desire to be heard. Being seen was a start.

THE 1960S: PROTESTS AND REBELLIOUS HAIRSTYLES

Across the Western world, economies began to flourish once more. Washing machines, vacuum cleaners and other instruments of domestic bliss had been furnished to homes during the 1950s, and now consumers had disposable incomes and a restlessness for new ideas. Televisions and radios helped to generate new myths, new needs and to challenge outdated traditions. In northern Europe and the United States, the classic concept of male and female roles came under fire: masculinity was variously and venomously attacked. That's not to say old-fashioned tropes disappeared completely: the 1960s saw James Bond brought to the screen by Sean Connery, starting with *Dr No* (1962), sporting a classic Madison Avenue cut. Italy preserved and refined its notion of the charming, elegant patriarch, attentive to detail. This classic, glamorous ideal still looked great in fashion and on film, even if it was out of step with changing times.

By the mid-1960s, the English-speaking world was assertively proposing new models through pop music and the press. When The Beatles arrived in New York in 1964, it was their long Mop Tops that caught the media's attention, not the music. They went on to become the world's biggest pop stars. Gradually, hair grew longer and longer. Literally.

In the language of style, the bohemian's disorderly appearance proclaimed his nonconformism; he professed not to care for his looks, to a level inversely proportional to his level of creativity and exuberance. (In reality, creating the boho look took as much time and attention as any other, including the sharp Mod or the greased Rockabilly.) Those who wanted to express their individuality by refusing any kind of aesthetic constriction shunned the barber and his razors, scissors, shaving creams and hairsprays,

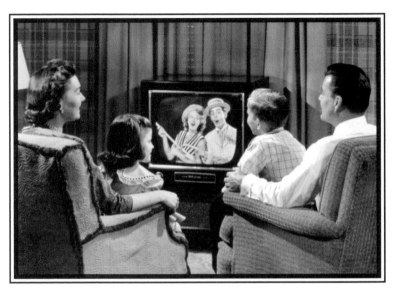

A family gathered around the television, 1950s

leaving hair free to grow with no restrictions. Young men adopted an androgynous hairstyle, choosing not to mark their gender difference and thereby challenging its relevance.

This wound some people up. In London, a subculture was developing that saw the rise of the Hippie, androgyny and multiculturalism as a warning of imminent societal apocalypse. Skinheads had been around as an offshoot of the Mods, listening to bands on the ska scene who played the rhythms of reggae music; now the severe haircut was adopted as a badge of membership by young working-class men who began to organize themselves into pseudo-military gangs. In 1969 they attacked members of the Pakistani community.

In France, the sense of frustration among young people was at a lack of change, at a government still pushing capitalist and consumerist ideas. In May 1968 students and workers voiced their frustration, ultimately bringing about socialist change that resonates today. Paris had been the hotspot for crazy Artist haircuts for decades — famously, Marcel Duchamp had a star shaved into the back of his head in 1921 — and now a new style flourished in the blasé intellectual, a naturally cosmopolitan and sensual man, constantly searching for novel modes of expression.

Everywhere there was a certain level of unrest among ethnic minorities, but it was in the United

States that unrest most famously boiled to the surface. African Americans, encouraged by new civil rights legislation and leaders such as Martin Luther King, started to reconsider and celebrate their own cultural specificity. One of the most visible markers was their hair, subjected to the Caucasian ideology of flatness and straightness for decades. Freedom meant free hair, and the Afro became a marker of pride and identity.

Over in London, Jimi Hendrix's white bandmates in The Experience showed their solidarity by adopting the style themselves (doubtless the result of hours of backcombing and industrial quantities of hairspray). The atmosphere of choice and freedom spread to other social minorities, and the word became liberation.

In this explosive setting, in which everything was questioned, hair provided a universal medium to represent visible change. In everyday life, manhood could take on divergent and multiple codes and meanings. A man could have curly, long, dyed, blow-dried hair, or wear streaked, braided, shaved, scented or stuck-to-the-head hair. From the 1960s onwards, nothing was ever the same. The men of the world had reclaimed the power of their hair for themselves.

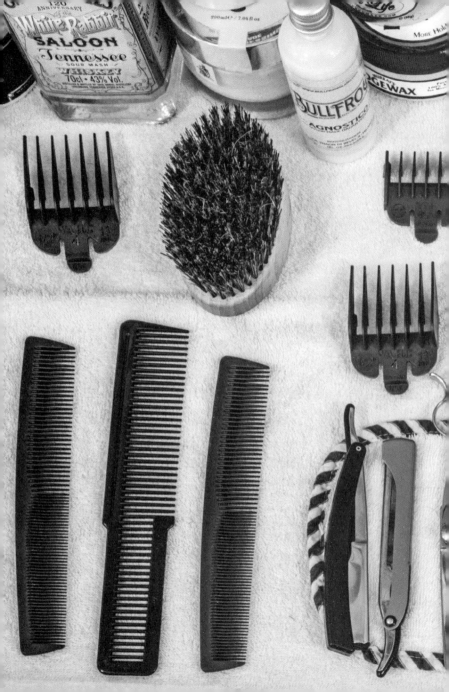

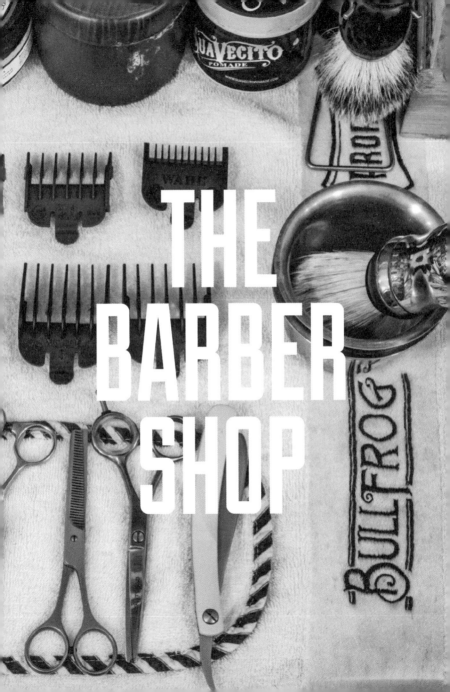

THE
BARBER
SHOP

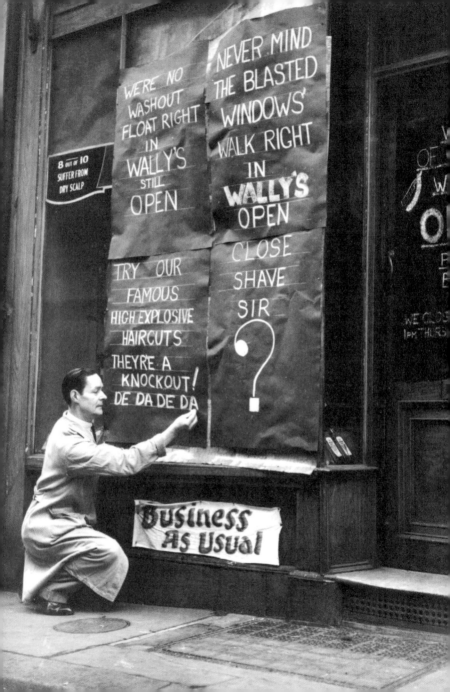

The barber shop is a bastion of masculinity, a place of ritual and sociability. Inside its doors, the barber serves as confidant and confessor, a master of elegance in whose hands men place their trust as well as their hair.

Traditionally, a barber would have some limited medical knowledge (the red-and-white striped pole of the barber-surgeon symbolizing blood and bandaging), which set him apart from his fellow men. This, in combination with his skill and dexterity with hair — in countless religious legends the symbolic store of strength, viz. Samson, Sikhism, the Mokawk tribes (see pp. 64–73), gave the barber a mystical aura: his tools were the sharp weapons of the shaman. In more recent times, the first shave in a barber's chair marked a milestone in a man's life, another stage in the passage from childhood to adulthood, like saying goodbye to short trousers, or completing National Service. Entering the barber shop was an initiation into a place reserved exclusively for men, where women were not admitted: a club.

Until well into the 1950s, the men of Britain and Europe kept weekly appointments at the barber's. There, they could indulge in sensuality, taking a journey of olfactory and emotional dimensions, of lotions and potions, of talcum powder, crystals and hot towels. However, things had already started to change radically in the United States. A puritan culture took hold that frowned on overt male grooming. The electric razor (patented as early as the 1900s but first successfully manufactured in 1931) became a common appliance in every home, removing the element of danger inherent in shaving with a cut-throat razor, and the ritual of going to the barber shop became less and less of a necessity. But, perhaps surprisingly, the greatest impact was brought about by the internal combustion engine. By the end of the 1940s car ownership was booming. City plans were being redesigned that capitalized on this new freedom for the workforce, in cleaner, lower-density housing with parks and gardens, and the suburbs began to sprawl. City centres that were crowded during working hours were now deserted in the evenings and much of the social life within them died. Just like the launderers and the shoe shiners, the barbers were forced to move elsewhere to continue their trade. In the halls of grand railway hotels, for example, they offered a quick shave to the new breed of businessmen, the commuters, on their way into or back from work.

During the 1960s, as young people on both sides of the Atlantic and around the Mediterranean differentiated themselves from their parents, the barber's style was seen as old-fashioned, and the trade fell into a period of deeper crisis. A major revolution took place in Swinging London: men started to go to women's hair salons without fearing for their masculinity. Hairdressers such as Vidal

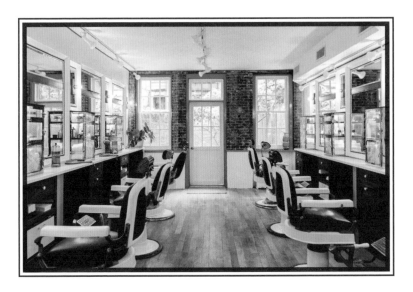

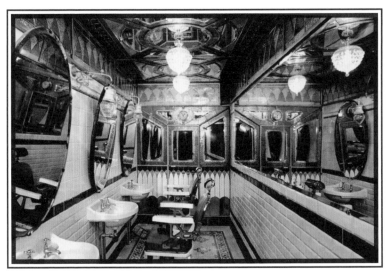

Top: Fellow Barber salon in Soho, New York. *Bottom:* Antica Barberia Giacalone, Genoa
Previous spread: Wally's barber shop after the London Blitz, 1940

Sassoon introduced unisex cuts (such as the famous geometric 'five points') and became the new darlings of a system that celebrated professions involved in show business and image creation.

But the barber shop never went away. During the lean years the immigrant communities — particularly Afro-Caribbean, Latino and Italian American — who lived in the urban outskirts of Western cities continued to regard life on the streets as a key component of their social life. For them, the barber shop constituted a primary place of encounter and sharing. Fashion and styles change and barber shops became popular again at the end of the 1990s. They attracted a clientele of men who wished to differentiate themselves from the masses by wearing a hairstyle that, in spite of being inspired by a classic cut, still appeared resolutely modern. The surge of interest in male grooming and the revival of a gentry look led to a veritable barber's shop renaissance in recent years. Fashionable establishments with old-school barber's chairs and vintage tools flourish all around the world in order to keep up with the demand. The contemporary barber shop now offers, once again, an experience exclusively tailored to men. Scents, shapes and labels conjure a universe that had almost disappeared, where without rush or fuss a man can spend guilt-free time on himself in the company of his peers.

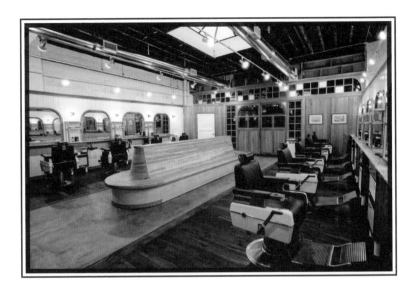

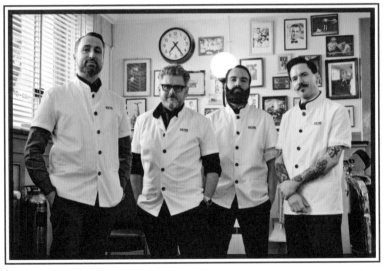

Top: Fellow Barber salon in Brooklyn, New York. *Bottom:* Staff of the New York Barbershop in Rotterdam, 'Best International Barbershop of the Year', 2013

CREW CUT

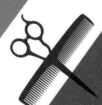

Popular among the rowing teams or 'crews' of
the Ivy League colleges from the 1930s, the Crew Cut
gained mainstream appeal during World War II
as the cut of choice in the United States military.
Millions of young recruits were enlisted and promptly
given this particularly short haircut.

The US Navy had imposed rules for beard and hair
length from its earliest days — logical hygiene
requirements based on the limited living space in
ships. During World War I, the short hairstyles sported
by the German army impressed US naval commanders
who copied the look for their own personnel. Apart
from practical cleanliness, extremely short hair and
a clean-shaven face also had the advantage of
unifying the appearance of a body of men, and
the Crew Cut soon became part of troop regulation
grooming standards for other military corps.
Its popularity outside the military was was fuelled
by these patriotic associations. The heroic figure
of the US Marine replaced the cowboy as a new role
model for American boys, who styled themselves
after GI Joe (the toy was first released in 1964).

At the end of World War II, the United States stood
reborn as the most powerful country on earth, with
a strong image to promote. Simple and no-frills,
the Crew Cut became the most popular haircut of the
1950s, emblematic of the clean and tidy American

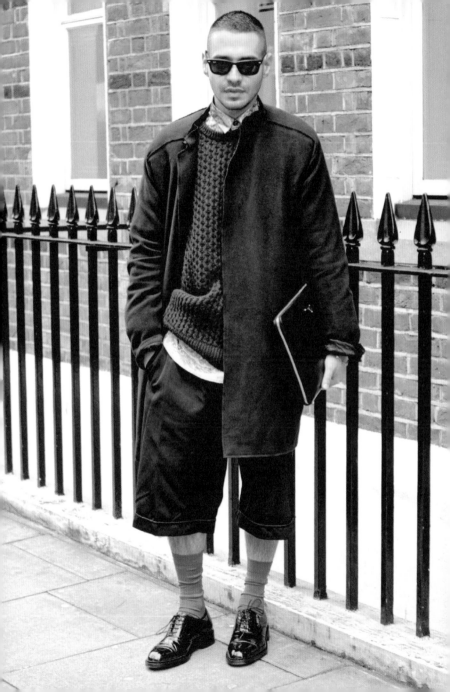

Way of Life. The classic US version of the Crew Cut is rather short all over the head, apart from the upper frontal section, which is left slightly longer to be combed to the side or raised. In time, many other versions developed, with varying lengths at the top and at the sides.

Outside the United States, this military cut was not particularly successful, perhaps seen as too harsh or too specifically American, and was generally interpreted as a cut at a unified length all over the head. Among the most famous men of the time to sport a Crew Cut were the saxophonist Gerry Mulligan and legendary actor Steve McQueen.

Saxophonist Gerry Mulligan playing at the Ridge Crest Inn, Rochester, c. 1958
Previous spread: A modern Crew Cut on the streets of London, 2013

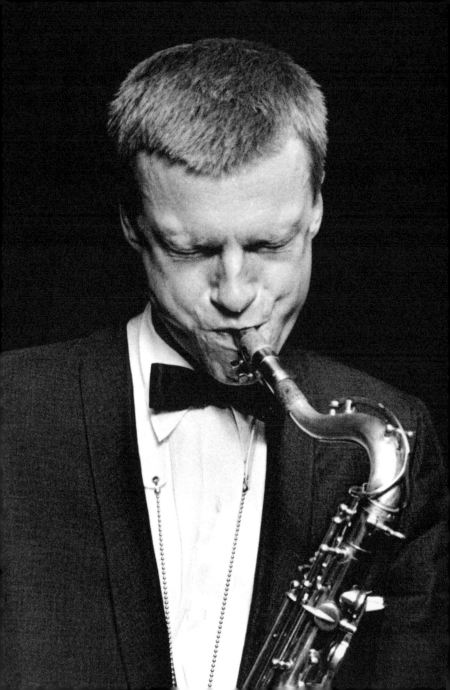

Do it yourself

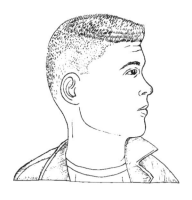

The hair is cut with clippers, starting from the sides, in a progressive tapering that can start at skin level

—

The back is treated similarly, with the taper even crossing the line of the occipital bone (approximately eye level)

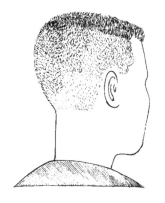

Next, the top is dried and combed upwards, sometimes using hairspray for hold; the comb and the clippers are then used together to create a uniform length, the perfect 'lawn'

Total look

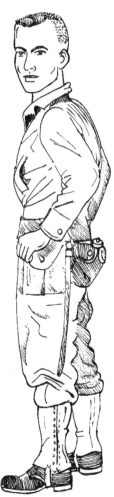

The Crew Cut requires constant reshaping in order to look consistently sharp and well-maintained

This short military hairstyle prevented hair from getting trapped inside a helmet or caught in a shirt collar — perfect for an active lifestyle

Outside the military field, this neat and versatile cut looks great when worn with formal clothing or with casual sportswear

COMPLETE THE LOOK

with gabardine service trousers, a khaki long-sleeved cotton shirt, military tattoos and dog tags

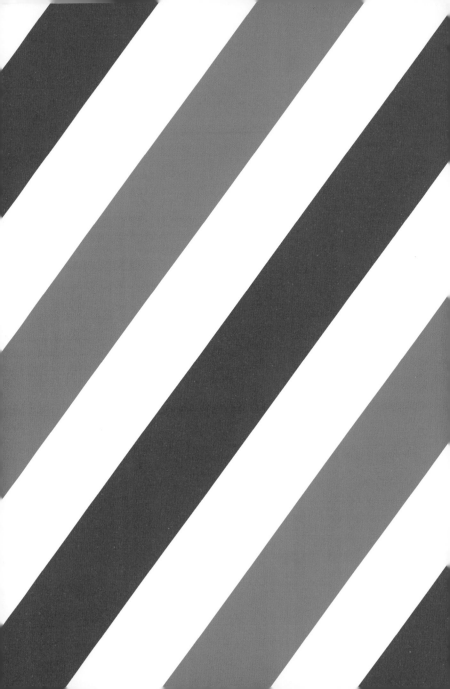

BRYLCREEM LOOK

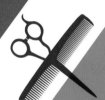

In the history of men's haircare, Brylcreem is an icon of Western culture: one of the earliest and best-known branded products. Surviving largely unchanged through wars, trends and social changes, the pomade has witnessed the evolution of hairstyles since 1928, when Birmingham's County Chemicals Company first introduced it to the consumer as Elite Hair Dressing Cream. Its formula was groundbreaking: part cream, part brilliantine, it kept hair in place and also made it shine. It was so good, the British government gave it an official stamp of approval during World War II, making Brylcreem standard issue in every soldier's kit bag.

The Royal Air Force (RAF), established in 1918, was the newest of the military forces. It developed a relatively modern culture and ethical code, along with a unique style, not just in uniforms and decorations. Pilots in particular were well aware of their glamour and status as members of a completely new breed of fighter, using the most sophisticated cutting-edge techniques and equipment. The RAF was popular for its unusually meritocratic attitude, a force open to whoever proved to have the skills and the ability to fly an aircraft, fix an engine or operate a control tower. Members of the lower-middle class found an alternative to a career as a clerk, a salesperson or an employee; even Black African and Caribbean conscripts from the wider reaches of the British

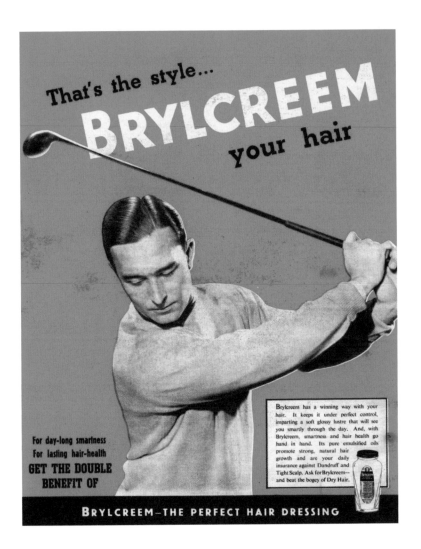

Advertisement for Brylcreem, c. 1950

Empire could join. These freedoms that distinguished the RAF from its older counterparts on land and sea, steeped in formality and tradition, were also reflected in the more relaxed rules for pilots' haircuts. Aviators were not obliged to cut their hair short, and were given the nickname 'the long-haired boys' by those who lacked the advantage off duty and out with girls.

An aviator had to go through all the Brylcreem in his personal kit if he wanted to keep his long hair in place during aggressive air battles in the German skies and these 'Brylcreem Boys' were idolized as dashing heroes. Looking sophisticated and well groomed in their light-blue, freshly ironed uniforms, the 'riff-raff' even dared defy the rules, leaving the top buttons of their jackets undone to wear silk scarves or – better still – the stockings of Moulin Rouge dancers tied around their necks.

Model sporting the Brylcreem look in Florence, 2014

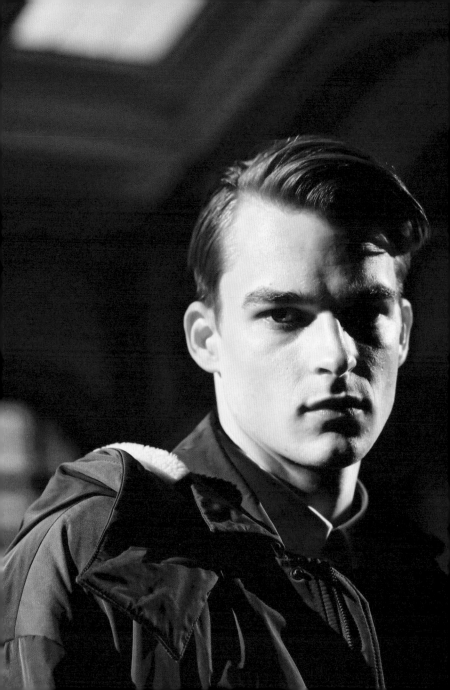

Do it yourself

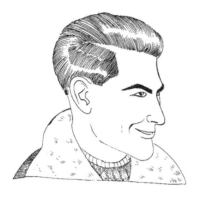

Brylcreem was used to
create the classic haircuts
of the 1930s and 1940s
(such as the Executive
Contour and Slick Back)
—
These hairstyles require
the hair to be combed to the
side, downwards or slightly
to the back, with a parting on
the side (usually the left)
and the shorter side naturally
blending with the tapering

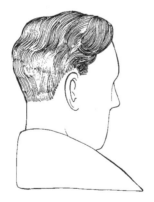

The crown is left longer and
can be softly styled

Total look

Glamorous aviators in the early twentieth century used large quantities of Brylcreem to keep their hair in place during flights

The style is now synonymous with the classic blue RAF service uniform

COMPLETE THE LOOK

with a vintage waistcoat, trousers tucked into black leather flying boots with sheepskin trim and the top button of a shirt left undone to reveal a delicate silk scarf

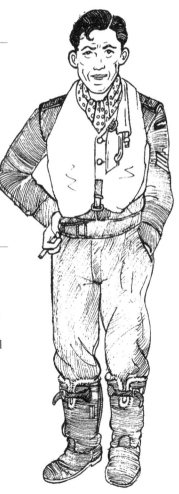

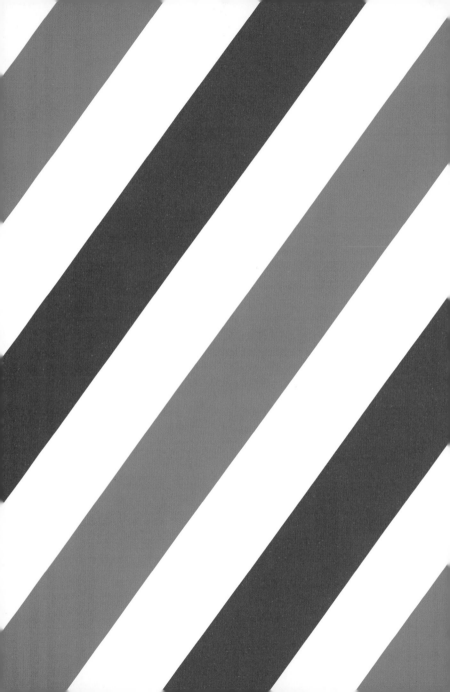

UNDERCUT

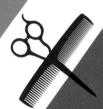

The Undercut, which reached the height of fashion across northern Europe in the 1930s, was the choice of young British sportsmen at the turn of the twentieth century. It was particularly popular with those involved in contact sports such as rugby. As an alternative to the King Edward VII (long on top, bushy sideburns, moustache and beard preferred), the cut was appreciated for its clean lines and practical, low-maintenance quality. In its native land — the German Empire, ruled by Prussian kings — it was commonly known as *der Inselhaarschnitt* (the island cut), because the long lock of hair sitting on top of the shaved head looked like a small patch of land surrounded by water. The hairstyle also took root with street gangs such as Birmingham's Peaky Blinders and crossed the Atlantic with Scottish and Irish working-class emigrants on their way to the United States.

The men of Hitler's army made this 'schizophrenic' haircut their own. Soldiers could show the clean-shaven sides and back and keep their longer hair on top hidden under a hat, side cap or helmet, combed back with brilliantine or Vaseline. Although there were minor variations to the cut, most common among the Wehrmacht was to have the hair on the neck entirely shaved (although three millimetres was the recommended length) and the longer hair cut high off the ears and shirt collar.

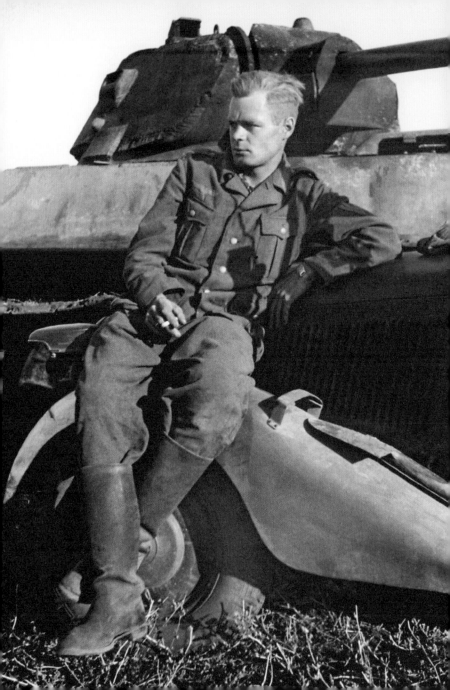

This haircut was chosen to express the Third Reich's bond with the glorious, belligerent past of Germany. Adopting the style of the Prussian Army, which enjoyed military successes during the eighteenth and nineteenth centuries, provided a nostalgic visual link that could be extended even further, towards Teutonic mythology. The plan of Germanic renaissance thus also included the revival of a hairstyle.

In Europe, perception of the Undercut changed when directly connected to the violence of invasion, and it was thereafter seen as a menacing style. US troops called it the 'whitewall', referring to the very white shaved scalp topped by darker hair, resembling the two-tone tyres popular on cars at the time.

In the early 1980s bands on the alternative and electro-synth scene started to wear the Undercut. David Bowie was an early adopter, sporting the look in the 1977 film *The Man Who Fell to Earth*. Left uncombed to hang loose, in the 1990s it evolved further when combined with longer curtains.

Model sporting the modern Undercut with a beard. *Previous spread:* German soldier on the Eastern Front, 1942

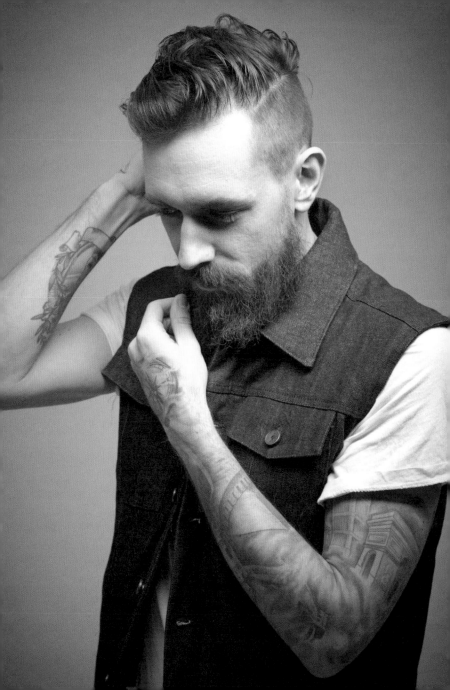

Do it yourself

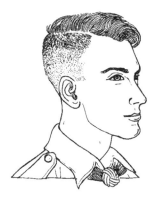

The peculiarity of this cut resides in the kind of tapering it requires

—

The hair is shaved with a straight razor up to two fingers above ear level and then tapered from skin level to three millimetres

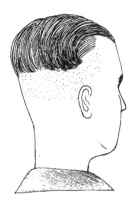

The top part is worn to the side or combed backwards. The cut is kept in place with the use of Brylcreem

Total look

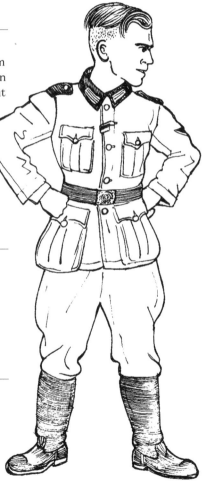

First sported by gangs in Birmingham in the early twentieth century and then the Wehrmacht soldiers, the Undercut is now a popular look on the streets of East London and Brooklyn

Today, men opt for the Undercut for its simplicity and the number of variations it presents

COMPLETE THE LOOK

with well-groomed stubble or a full beard. For outfit inspiration look no further than the latest urban fashion magazines

Try wearing a hat to conceal the longer hair on top and reveal only the closely shaven sides for a totally different style

55

ZOOT SUITER

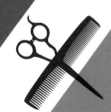

The Zoot Suiters had an obsessive attitude towards their hair. The clothing may have taken the glory in fashion history, but the subculture's exuberant hairstyle was its soul: long quiffs daubed with brilliantine, bouncing and flapping on the men's foreheads as they danced uninhibited in underground jazz clubs, scandalizing puritan culture.

Emerging from the African American jazz scene of 1930s' New York, the look spread among Italian Americans to Chicago and the East Coast of the United States, and was embraced as their own by Mexican immigrants living in Los Angeles, who called themselves Pachucos. Wearing the Zoot Suit showed allegiance to a group that would dictate its own style, a stand against the tyranny of a fashion world accessible only to the elite few. Its appeal was taken up, not just by immigrants, but also by young working-class youths looking for a group identity.

Along the way it picked up various unsavoury associations of gangsterism from its popularity with nightclub owners and the Mob. The feathered hats and the extremely long watch chains all became synonymous with illegality. Exuberant Latino Zoot Suiters formed one of the first markedly 'foreign' subcultures to affirm itself in US society, an ethnic minority staking its claim to an overtly separate American identity; greasy and coated with pomade,

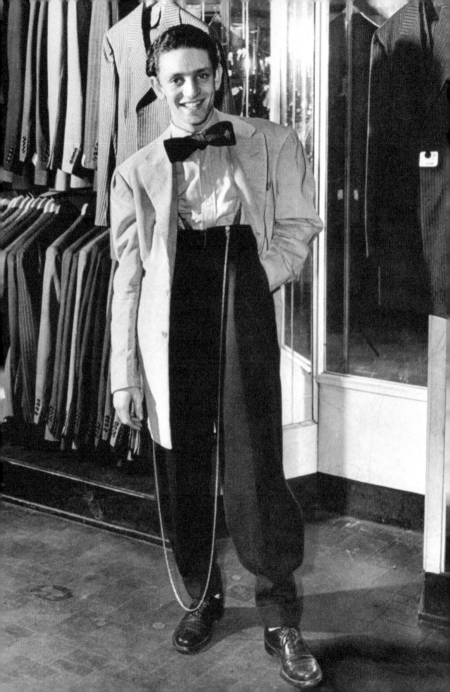

their hair was one of the strongest ethnic symbols in Latin culture.

These were the days before ready-to-wear: young men would have their suits made up by local tailors, instructing them to follow the extreme lines of the cut. Jackets were broad across the shoulders, tailored to the fingertips and reaching to the knees; trousers were tight around the high waist before ballooning out at the knee, dramatically tapering back to the ankle. Jim Carrey wore a Zoot Suit in *The Mask* (1994): bright, bold and baggy.

During World War II the vast amounts of material required placed the Zoot Suiters at odds with clothes rationing. Their outfits were pounced upon as emblematic of an 'un-American' culture, for propping up a black market in wool. The Zoot Suit Riots of 1943 pitted US servicemen against Mexican American Zoot Suiters on the streets of Los Angeles. When caught, the standard treatment for Zoot Suiters was to have their clothes ripped off and burnt or torn to pieces. Hair was shaved off completely. All this took place in public, on the spot where the Zoot Suiter had been stopped. The atmosphere of racial and sartorial tension was captured in the 1981 film *Zoot Suit*. Amazingly, nobody died, but a law was passed banning the style in public.

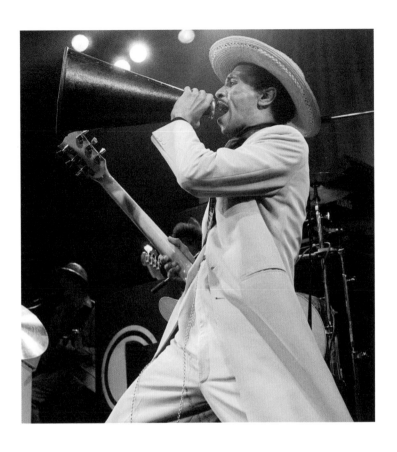

Kid Creole (August Darnell) performing on stage, United Kingdom, 1982
Previous spread: Jerome Mendelson modelling a Zoot Suit in a clothing store, 1942

Do it yourself

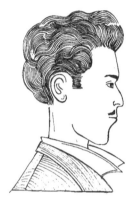

A long haircut, for wavy hair

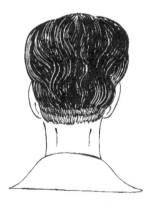

The sides and back are
slightly tapered and
the top lengths are brought
to the back with plenty
of Brylcreem

Total look

This exuberant look originated in New York's jazz clubs in the 1930s — the shiny long quiff was perfect for bouncing along wildly to the popular music of the time

COMPLETE THE LOOK

with a bright and baggy tailor-made suit, high-waisted trousers and pointed shoes with an oversized bow tie

Perfect your eccentric outfit with a long metallic keychain sticking out from the knee-length jacket and a broad-rimmed, flat hat

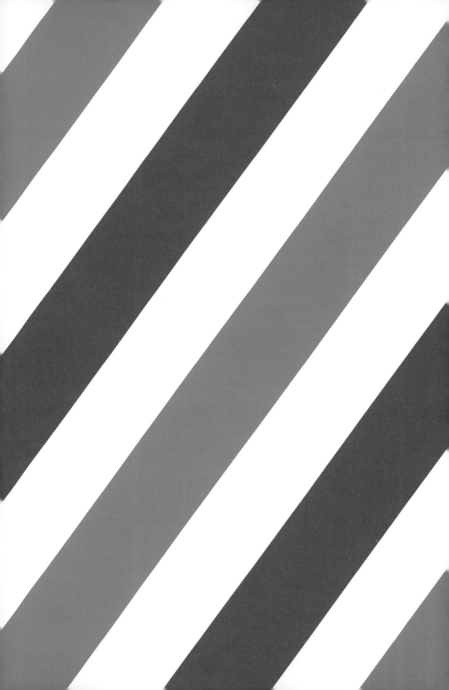

MOHAWK

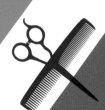

This haircut has its origins among the Native American peoples of the Iroquois League who lived in the large forests of the northeastern United States. These included the Mohawks. Fierce Mohawk warriors shaved the sides of their heads, leaving only a brush-like strip of hair at the top, running straight from the forehead to the nape, which was kept stiff with boar grease or resin. Hair was used as an instrument to intimidate the enemy, to provoke and defy rivals in a culture that routinely scalped its victims. Indeed, the Iroquois nations believed that a man's strength resided in his hair.

The Last of the Mohicans, a cult book in American literature, has contributed to the heroic appeal of Native American styles. This historical novel of 1826 conveyed an image of the Native American as a righteous fighter of mythical power that endured in popular culture throughout the twentieth century.

During World War II, the Screaming Eagles (the US paratrooper division sent to Normandy) took advantage of this perception, adopting the instantly recognizable symbol. Inspired by one Native paratrooper, this group of soldiers broke military rules, transforming their hair into Mohawks and painting their faces with tribal signs.

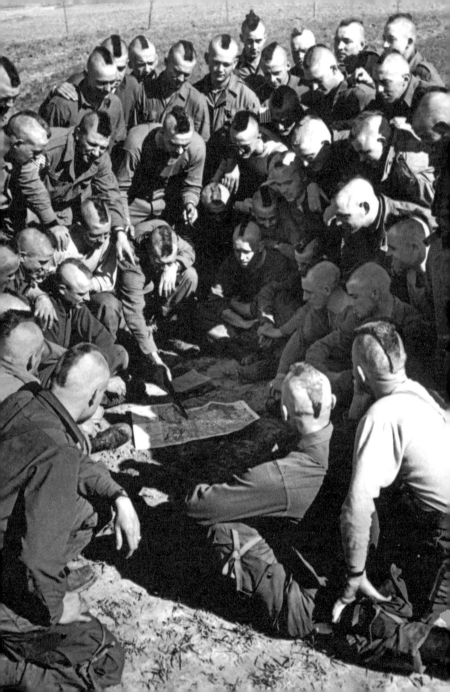

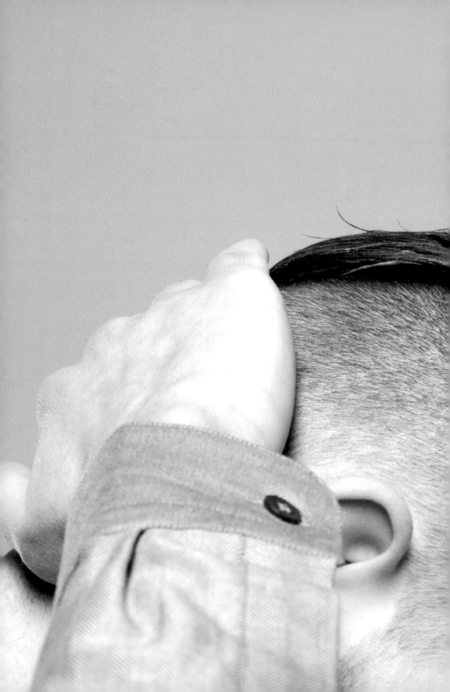

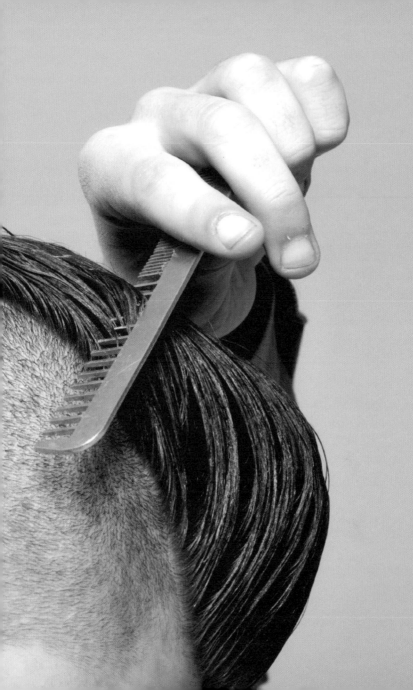

The echo of the merciless Iroquois warriors ready to scalp the enemy resounded in the United States and across Germany too. Not yet regarded as an oppressed population (which came later, in the progressive 1960s), Native Americans were still perceived as a dangerous enemy, savagely expert in the art of war. Photographs of the Screaming Eagles were published on the pages of *Stars and Stripes* military magazine and spread all over the world, presenting the soldiers as the natural heirs to ancient and heroic courage.

The Mohawk haircut resurfaced during the 1950s and 1960s, when it was the haircut of choice of US special corps fighting the Korean and Vietnam Wars. It is visual shorthand on film: in Martin Scorsese's *Taxi Driver* (1976), Robert De Niro's Mohawk served as an indicator of his declaration of war on society. The haircut and its variant the Mohican (characterized by longer stiff, upright spikes and lurid dyes) symbolized the same alienation when they were embraced by the Punk bands of London and New York in the 1970s and Hardcore bands of California during the 1980s.

British Punk with tattoos, piercings and Mohawk, 1982. *Page 67*: US paratroopers preparing for a mission, Arras, France, 1945

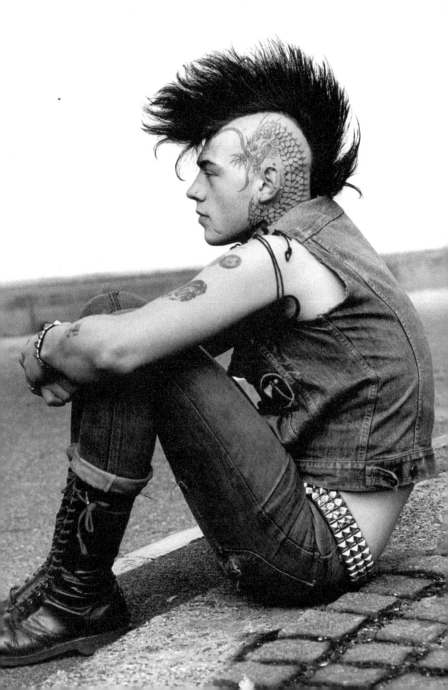

Do it yourself

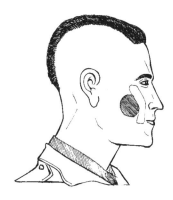

Hair is cut short, in a three-fingers-wide section at the front, ending in a point at the back of the head

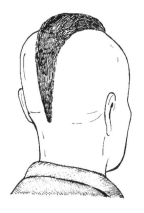

The sides are fully shaved to the skin, and remaining hair is styled straight up to give a brush-like appearance, using hairspray to make it stand away from the head in longer styles

Total look

Along with tribal war paint, the original fierce Mohawk hairstyle was designed to intimidate

During the 1970s, the cut was adopted and customized by Punks, who styled it upright with strong gel or even glue

Today's anti-materialistic and nonconformist Punk embraces all types of clothes and accessories, any combination of textures and colours

COMPLETE THE LOOK

with a black leather jacket, a plain shirt, baggy work trousers and heavy industrial boots

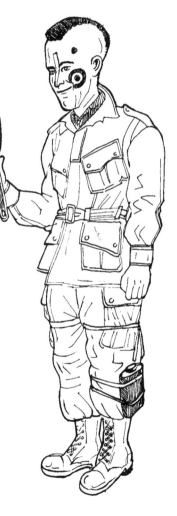

SLICK BACK

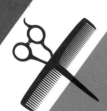

Long hair combed back over the head and kept in place by layers of pomade, grease or brilliantine has been a symbol of masculine elegance since the 1910s. The Slick Back style was designed to preserve the vigour and strength of the hair while holding it in place in a shiny, unified shape. Promoters included Italian showman Rudolph Valentino and Hollywood star Clark Gable, who amplified its appeal during the 1920s and 1930s. It was the choice of the seductive man *par excellence*, the mark of sex appeal in high society.

It is interesting to note that, although the Slick Back was not considered a product of Anglo-American culture, this hairstyle was hugely popular in the United States. There, the perceived sensual superiority of Mediterranean men was proudly expressed by Italian immigrants and widely emulated by others who wore their hair shiny and sleek.

A highly effective weapon of seduction, it was embraced by Hollywood, thus influencing moviegoers around the world. Bela Lugosi wore it as the titular antihero in *Count Dracula* (1931); Gable as Rhett Butler in *Gone with the Wind* (1939). Sportsmen, actors and *bons vivants* all became fans of this emblematic hairstyle.

The cosmetics industry supported the trend, manufacturing products that became more and more

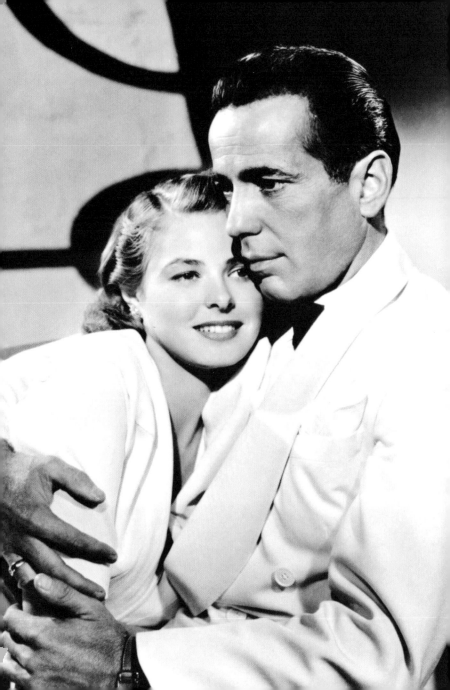

effective in straightening and subduing the hair.
Wealthier people could afford delicately scented
pomades, while the rest had to make do with edible
oils or, worse, with petrol.

The Slick Back was a hairstyle that admitted no
flaws, not a single hair out of place: what mattered
was the compact and smooth effect. For maintenance,
the hairstyle had to stay in place during the night.
The public image of the urbane and cultured man
attending high-society parties clashed with the
rather unattractive private reality of a man wearing
a hairnet in bed (or even a stocking, if he could not
afford the hairnet).

After falling out of fashion during the 1960s and 1970s,
when hair worn loose in the wind became all the
rage, the Slick Back reappeared in the 1980s among
New York stockbrokers, on David Bowie during
his Thin White Duke period and, sometime later,
on Johnny Depp.

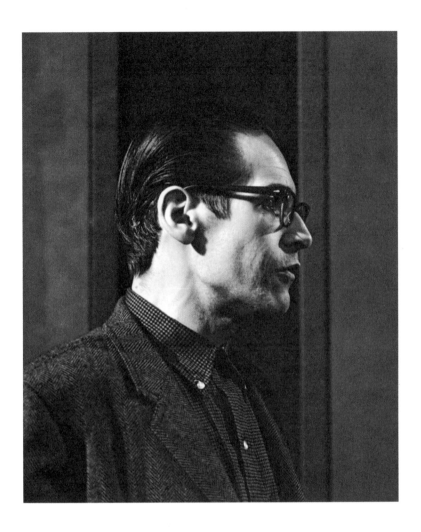

Jazz pianist Bill Evans, United Kingdom, 1965. *Previous spread:* Humphrey Bogart and Ingrid Bergman in the movie *Casablanca*, 1942

Do it yourself

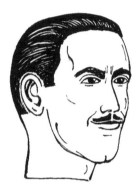

All the hair is combed backwards, where it is cut to a single, blunt length, usually at the nape of the neck

—

The front section needs to be left long enough to reach from the forehead over the top of the head and down the back, considerably longer than the sides, which are tapered and combed back to avoid excessive volume

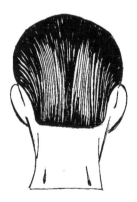

Plenty of Brylcreem is used to style the cut

Total look

The smooth Slick Back style,
a classic masculine and elegant look,
becomes even more sophisticated
when sported with a moustache

The hair must be kept smooth,
compact and in place twenty-four
hours a day, therefore it is advisable to
wear a hairnet or a stocking in bed
for protection

COMPLETE THE LOOK

with a three-piece, light-coloured,
pinstriped suit with a fancy tie and
leather brogues

Combine the Slick Back with the
Undercut for a contemporary twist
on two traditional hairstyles

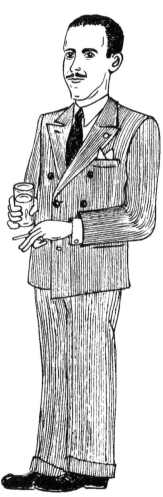

ITALIANO

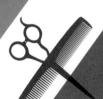

This haircut recalls a time when, for a few years in the mid-1950s, Italy was the centre of the cultural world. Hollywood and European royalty were found on the studio lots of Rome and at the couture shows at the Palazzo Pitti in Florence. The style speaks of sunshine and glamour, of Gregory Peck romancing Audrey Hepburn in the 1953 film *Roman Holiday*.

The so-called *bel paese* (beautiful country) retained a reputation for style and a taste for beauty untarnished by either World War II or the Fascism of Mussolini's regime. Post-war Italian Modernism acquired international prestige. As the economy recovered, the Italian artisan tradition was revived and translated into objects of an aesthetic quality that promised a totally new era. Italy is a country where being well dressed is not only a privilege but also a duty for both rich and poor; it became a paradigm of post-war elegance across social classes.

The example was seized upon by the British modernists, the Mods. Men's suits were slimmer in fit and jackets and trousers shorter, assuring comfort while driving a Vespa scooter. The look was synonymous with the laid-back approach to life that still today is associated with post-war Italy, exemplified by actor Marcello Mastroianni, star of *La Dolce Vita* (1960) and the embodiment of the charming and dapper Italian lover.

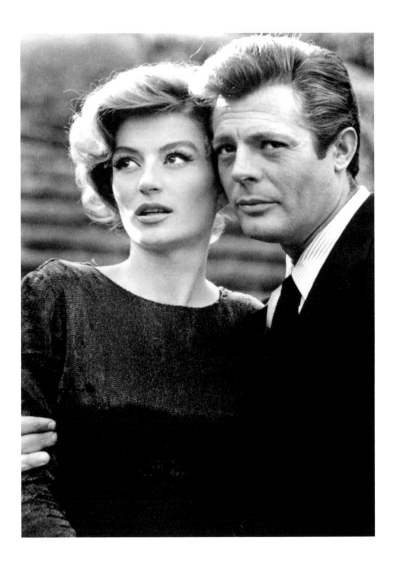

Marcello Mastroianni and Anouk Aimée in *La Dolce Vita*, 1960

Do it yourself

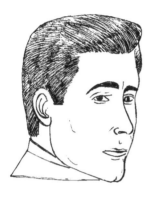

Like the Madison Avenue, the Italiano is an adaptation of the visibly parted Executive Contour, worn longer. Hair is cut with scissors rather than clippers or a razor

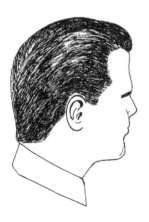

In its classic version, with a side parting, the hair is softly combed back and set slightly to the side in the top part. The haircut is to be styled only with hairdryer and brush: no product is needed

Total look

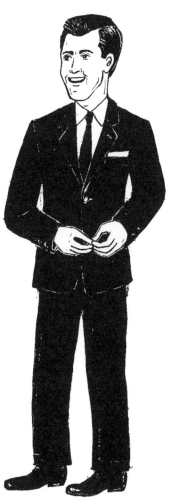

One doesn't need to be Italian to sport the dapper Italiano. This is a look suitable for any laid-back and refined gentleman

This haircut is much appreciated for its simplicity. It highlights the natural beauty of the hair by leaving it free from styling products

COMPLETE THE LOOK

with a trendy slim-fit suit — synonymous with Italian elegance and perfect for almost any occasion — and don't forget your Vespa, the ultimate accessory for your dolce vita style

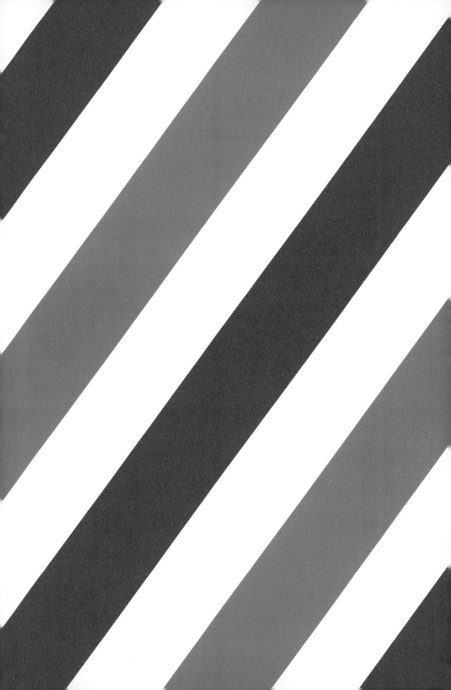

IVY LEAGUE

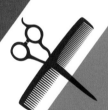

The Ivy League cut, a hairstyle synonymous
with American elegance, began as a mark of
sartorial rebellion. Since their foundation, the most
prestigious colleges of the East Coast – Harvard,
Yale, Pennsylvania, Princeton, Columbia, Brown,
Dartmouth and Cornell Universities – the Ivy League
had imposed strict dress and hairstyle codes.
Young gentlemen's hair had to be short and cut
frequently, ensuring all students had a fresh and
clean appearance, appropriate to businessmen in the
making. But in the can-do post-war atmosphere of
the 1950s, a new breed of student – the teenager
– attempted a reinterpretation of these formal rules.

In the new casual-yet-conservative campus look,
loafers, Argyle socks, tartan jackets and shirts
replaced the grey flannel suits worn by previous
generations. The haircut is simply a slightly longer
version of the Crew Cut, allowing greater freedom
in styling, though whether worn with a parting
or simply falling to the front, the hair is always still
neatly combed. It was the barbers who named this
cut the Ivy League (or sometimes, the Princeton).

The Ivy League cut spread across the continent,
becoming a must for all upper-middle-class
Americans – and any who aspired to join their ranks.
It was the look of relaxed entitlement, of the future
establishment, of the Kennedys. Hollywood was quick

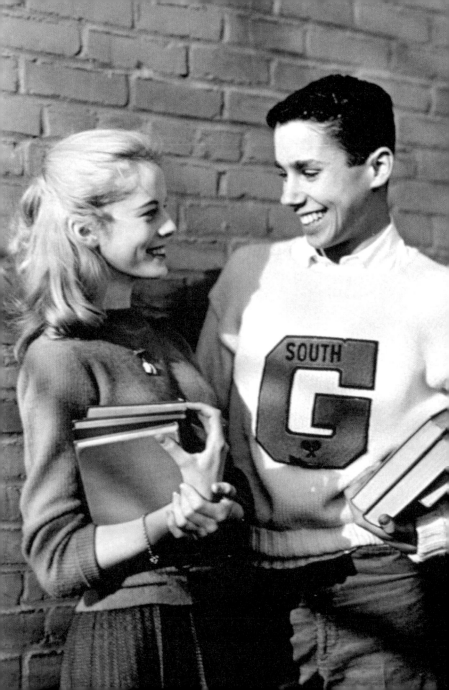

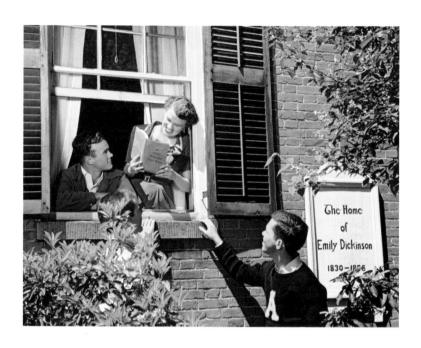

Ivy League students at the window of Emily Dickinson's home, Massachusetts, 1950
Previous spread: The varsity sweater with campus initials was a classic look of the 1950s

to use it to exemplify the lifestyle of this young elite, in movies such as 1959's *The Young Philadelphians*. Soon it proved to be one of those classic cuts that appear in the pictures hanging on the walls of every barber's shop.

With the exception of a few rare and daring Rockabilly quiffs, yearbooks from Yale, Dartmouth, Harvard, Princeton and the rest register the ubiquity of the Ivy League cut. It remained the prevalent college style for over a decade. However, following the 'Summer of Love' in 1967, even the most conservative universities started to register a change. Opening their doors to a more diverse student population meant that Hippies now mingled with the priviliged prep-school students who had been their natural clientele. Dress codes became less rigid under the influence of different cultures and trends, and a fashion for long hair created a style revolution on the campuses, spreading among students and academics alike: the Ivy League cut lived on as nostalgia.

Do it yourself

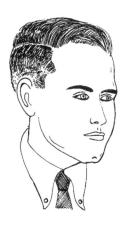

Short on the back and sides, the Ivy League can be cut in different lengths but is usually tapered quite short up to ear level

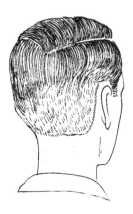

The hair on top of the head and at the upper sides is left slightly longer. Instead of Brylcreem, the haircut can also be styled with pomade

Total look

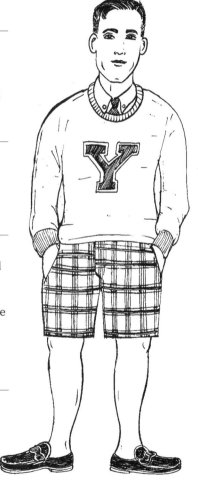

This neatly tapered cut is absolutely essential to the Ivy League look — a classic hairstyle, it is suitable for all men and never goes out of fashion

The Ivy League style was inspired by traditional British leisurewear in the 1950s

Tired of the conservative grey flannel suits prevalent at the time, college and high school students opted for rougher, more casual fabrics and were proud to display their hard-earned varsity letters or school patches on jackets or sweaters

COMPLETE THE LOOK

with a button-down Oxford shirt, a Shetland sweater, a sack jacket, penny loafers and argyle socks

95

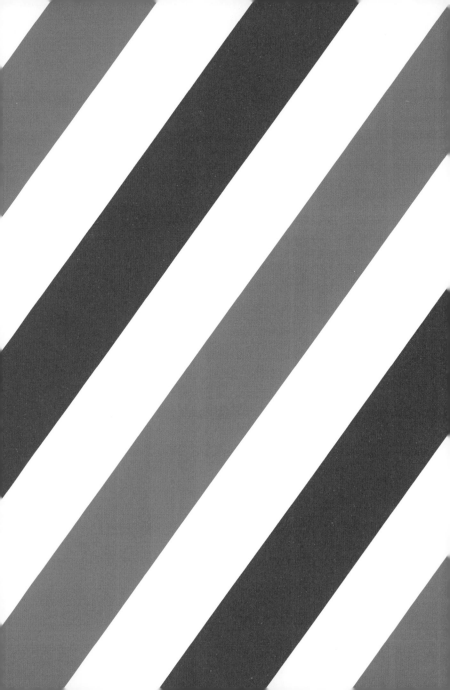

MADISON AVENUE

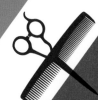

Madison Avenue in New York is where, during the 1950s, creative agencies gave birth to modern advertising: the eponymous haircut is instantly recognizable to viewers of the television series *Mad Men*. It is a city cut, slick and sophisticated, the badge of the successful self-made man who likes his cocktails Old-Fashioned.

These admen launched a global campaign promoting a new type of nuclear family that epitomized the American Dream. The male head of the household was accomplished and successful, a man who had beaten tough competition to 'make it' to his position in society; a husband and a father whose daily battle began every morning when he stepped out of his front door. He worked hard to make sure his family could afford its suburban house, filled with the latest consumer appliances and popular brands.

In fact this male archetype was largely a reflection of the professionals who devised him, striving to get ahead on Madison Avenue. This was the self-image that the United States exported all over the post-war world and to its own people: a nation of winners and consumers. Agencies such as Norman, Craig & Kummel contributed to the creation of a strong paradigm, the success of which was then assured by blanket media coverage. From radio jingles to magazines and television, advertising

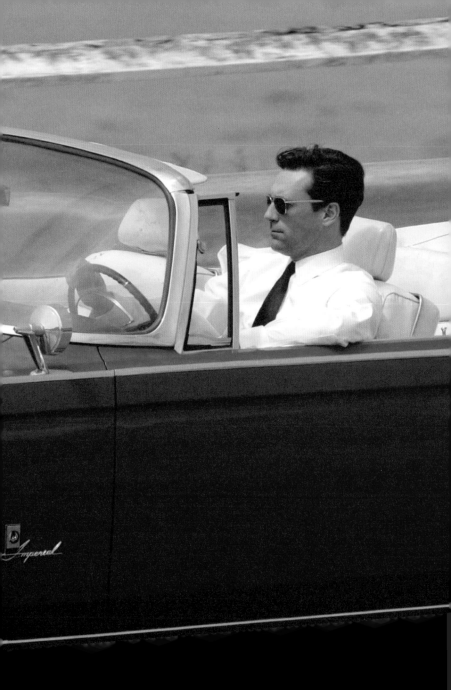

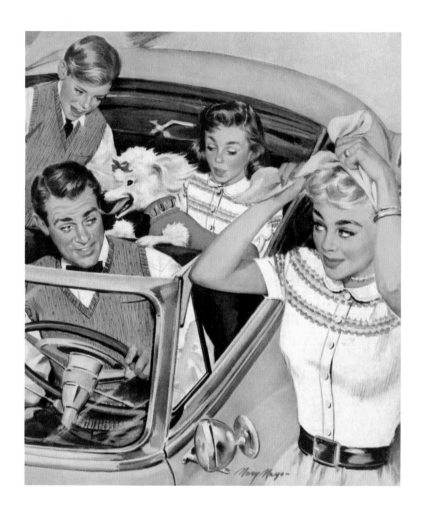

Advertisement for sweaters by the illustrator Mary Mayo, 1950s. *Previous spread:*
Actor Jon Hamm playing Don Draper in the television series *Mad Men*, San Pedro CA, 2010

campaigns invaded every home, driving the desires of American families.

The Madison Avenue man symbolized a society that appeared to have no limits in terms of expansion and the pursuit of wealth. His impeccable appearance only confirmed his success: roomy pinstriped suits, revealing nothing of his figure, proclaimed his mastery over nature and were the product of a modern ready-to-wear clothing industry, one in which Europe lagged behind. An integral part of the total look, the Madison Avenue cut was the democratic haircut that witnessed the passing of the hat age, and it was to play a leading role in male styling during the decades that followed. Although this cut did not need hair pomade or any other product, the Madison Avenue allowed some minor aesthetic individuality, thus fostering the creation of a niche market for men's beauty products and grooming.

Do it yourself

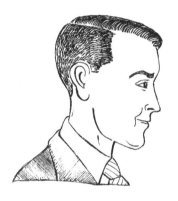

The Madison Avenue is an evolution of the earlier Executive Contour, a cut with a highly visible side parting. In this new hairstyle, the hair on top of the head is long and combed away from the parting while the sides and the nape are classically tapered

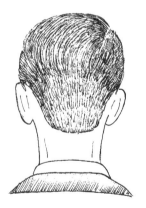

More length at the sides and at the top must follow the shape of the head without creating volume

Total look

Popularized by the incredibly successful television series *Mad Men*, this style is the epitome of the suave, sophisticated businessman look

A smart suit with thin lapels and tapered trousers, white button-down shirt and slim tie are still closely associated with New York elegance

COMPLETE THE LOOK

with a classic hat, teardrop-shaped aviator sunglasses and a leather briefcase. Oh, and an Old-Fashioned cocktail of course...

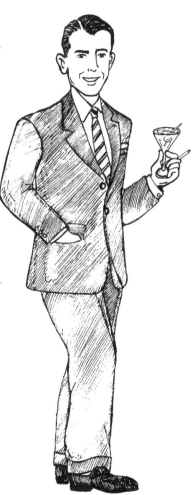

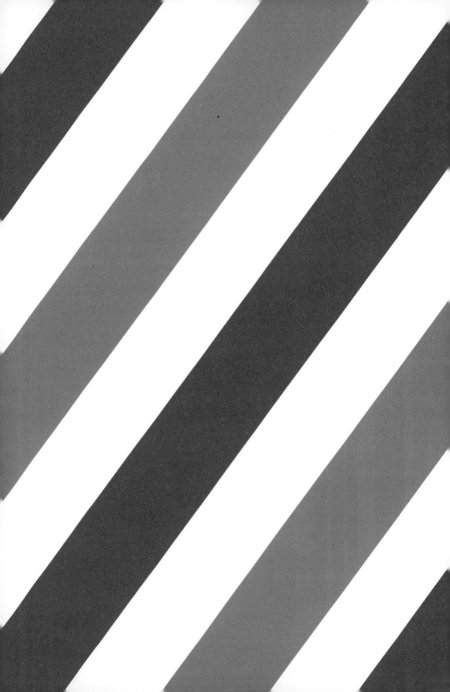

CAESAR

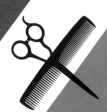

How ironic to be called 'hairy' when you suffer from hair loss. In trying to hide what people in ancient Rome considered a deformity, Caius Julius Caesar used to comb what hair he had left down towards his forehead, in a style that now bears his name. (The Latin *caesaries* is translated as 'hair'; *caesariatus*, bushy-haired, so the cognomen, or nickname, that was transferred down the line as an emperor's title might well have been humorous from the outset.)

Over two millennia, the Caesar has projected an image of power, worn by some of the greatest men in history. Whether it was down to the prevailing taste for Neoclassicism that emerged in the late eighteenth century or perhaps because of his own receding hairline, even the French Emperor Napoleon liked to comb his hair Julius Caesar style.

It was during the 1950s that the film industry staged a heroic comeback for this haircut in the modern age. The ideal of classical beauty and the neo-Roman look spread all over the world thanks to the Italian pepla movies of the Cinecittà studios, and the 'sword and sandal' Hollywood epics set in ancient Rome or Greece. From *Quo Vadis?* (1951) to *The Last Days of Pompeii* and *Ben-Hur* (both 1959), the Caesar haircut ruled as a noble model of elegance. The most famous interpretation of the cut was seen on Marlon Brando, playing Marc Antony in the film adaptation of

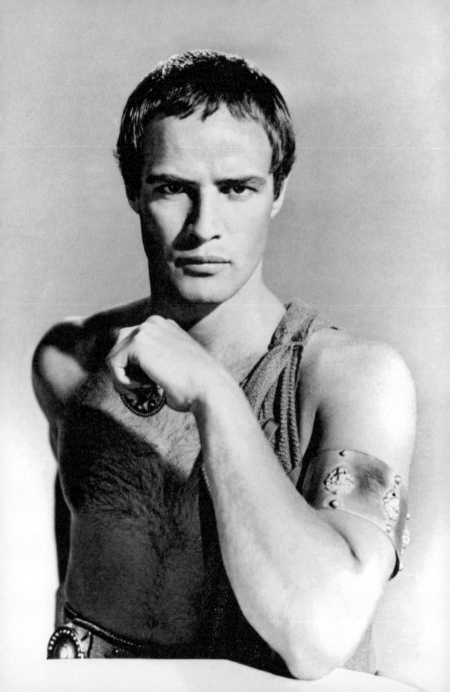

Shakespeare's *Julius Caesar* in 1953. The craze for classical adaptations also transferred to the stage, making this haircut very popular in London theatres and on Broadway. However, it remained largely the preserve of costume designers and the acting community. During the 1990s, the hairstyle enjoyed new popularity when adopted by famous Hollywood actors, George Clooney and Russell Crowe.

Model sporting a contemporary Caesar cut. *Previous spread*: American actor Marlon Brando as Mark Anthony in the movie *Julius Caesar*, 1953

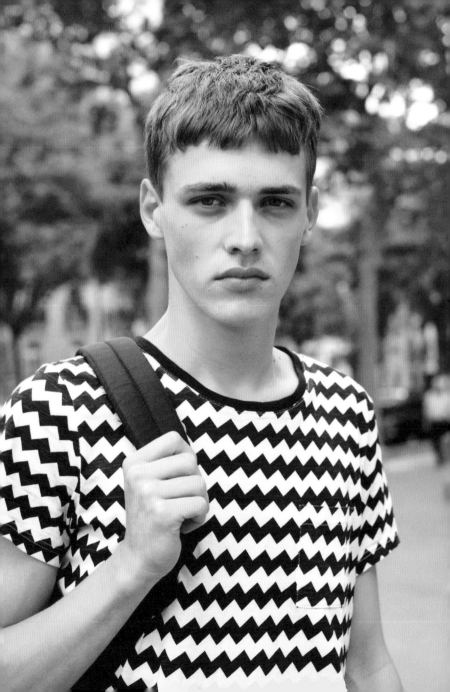

Do it yourself

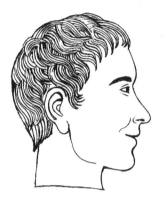

This medium-length cut follows the curve of the head.

—

Tapering radiates from a single spot at the back, near the crown, with hair combed to the front from the centre of the head

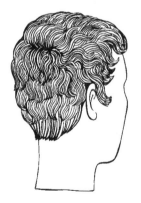

Hair can be left natural or styled with hair oil or wax

Total look

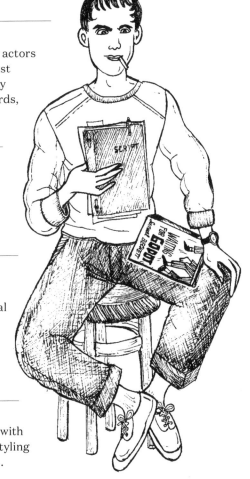

This look was popularized by actors
on the stages of London's West
End and New York's Broadway
who combed their hair forwards,
imitating classical statues

Inspired by Caesar himself,
this is a low-maintenance
hairstyle, perfect for
the more casual gentleman

COMPLETE THE LOOK

however you like: this imperial
style goes just as well with
a formal business suit
as with a pair of jeans and
canvas shoes

The short-cropped hairstyle with
a fringe is also an excellent styling
alternative for balding men…

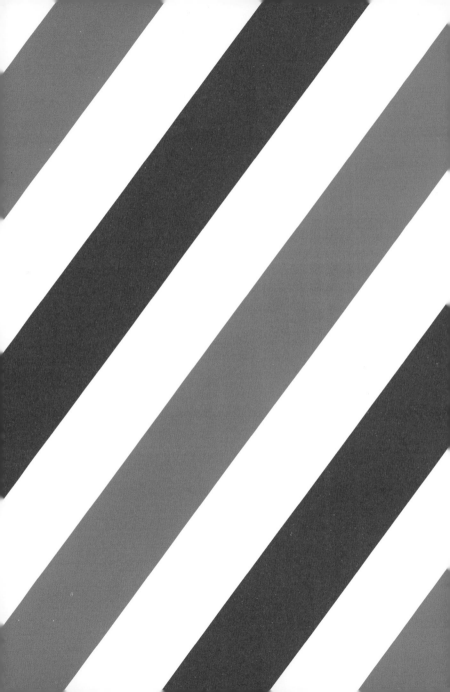

ROCKABILLY

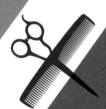

Rockabilly is the lovechild of rock 'n' roll and the country music of the southeastern United States, the unholy union of 'rock' and hill-'billy'. The style is one-part Elvis to two-parts Tennessee bumpkin: tattoos, bowling shirts, horn-rimmed glasses and a mane of greased-back hair.

The year 1954 was rock 'n' roll's year zero: for ever after, time would be divided into 'Before Elvis' and 'After Elvis'. The King's primal, sexually charged sound shook the United States like an earthquake, threatening to demolish the walls of cleanliness and control behind which its mainstream culture was hiding. (They'd all been listening to crooners like Bing Crosby and Patti Page. Page's ditty 'How Much Is That Doggie in the Window?' topped the charts in 1953 for more than two months.) Elvis Presley was a white man who sang black music, swinging his hips in the face of puritan restriction. He brought the energy of a discriminated minority straight into the nation's homes, to face the skeleton of racial segregation hanging in their cupboards.

Rock 'n' roll, epitomized by Elvis's flashy, dirty and pheromone-laden hairstyle, became the lifeblood of artistic generations to come, and its first offshoot was Rockabilly. The music was a rustic and raw interpretation, combining traditional Southern country with black music. Rockabilly icons included

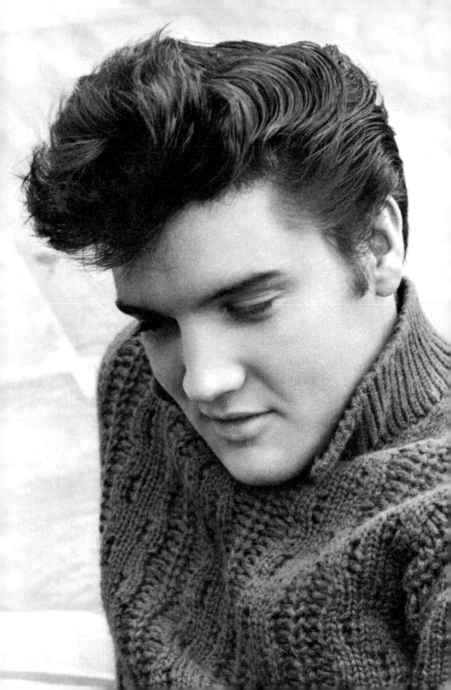

Buddy Holly, Gene Vincent, Eddie Cochran and Jerry Lee Lewis, stars who did not bother to sneeze into their hands but could not bear anyone stepping on their blue suede shoes — as Carl Perkins famously sang in 1956.

Rockabilly hairstyles echo Elvis's. There is not one specific cut, but the long length, enthusiastic use of brilliantine and big sculpted or curly quiffs are cornerstones of the look. A banana-shaped volume is completed at the nape by a 'duck's arse' (often euphemistically referred to as a 'DA'), a shape apparently invented by Philadelphia barber Joe Cirello in 1940 and later incorporated into other hairstyles including the one worn by Teddy Boys. Singer Mac Curtis wore a variant style: a Flat Top cut, front lock falling forwards, with sides combed back in a shape that clearly echoes the finned silhouette of the early 1950s' Eldorado Cadillac.

Rockabilly is essentially a US style, though it travelled internationally through the music scene. It was embraced again in Britain during the 1980s, when pop stars such as the Stray Cats and homegrown talents the Polecats led a revival; interest in the genre and its style endures today.

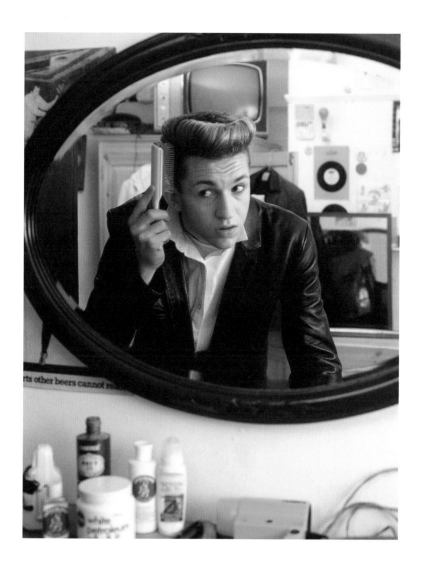

A member of the Polecats fixing his Rockabilly style, c. 1981. *Previous spread*: Elvis Presley, 1956.

Do it yourself

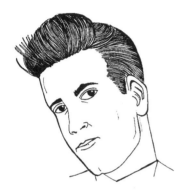

Hair is worn medium-long, cut to about ten centimetres. The front and top sections are shaped into a voluminous quiff that falls backwards softly. At the back, the hair is cut square on the neck

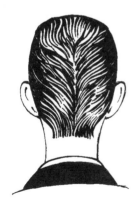

From both sides, the hair is combed backwards, integrated into the quiff at the top and meeting at the centre line down the back, forming a very short duck's arse. A comb is inserted into the centre of the back hair, pulling the two sides downwards. Heavy use of pomade keeps the look in place

Total look

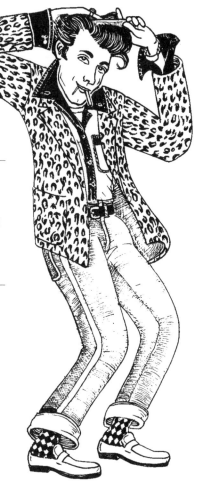

The Rockabilly's style
is the perfect blend between
Elvis Presley's rock 'n' roll
charisma and the more laid-back
vibes of Southern country music

The big sculpted, curly quiff is
perfectly complimented by a touch
of kitsch, such as a shirt embroidered
with diamonds or emblazoned with
animal prints

COMPLETE THE LOOK

with a bowling shirt, horn-rimmed
glasses, and of course, a pair
of (preferably blue) suede shoes

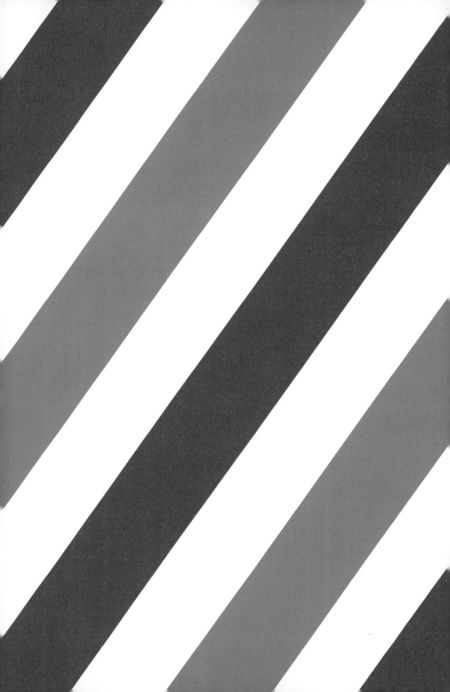

TEDDY BOY

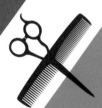

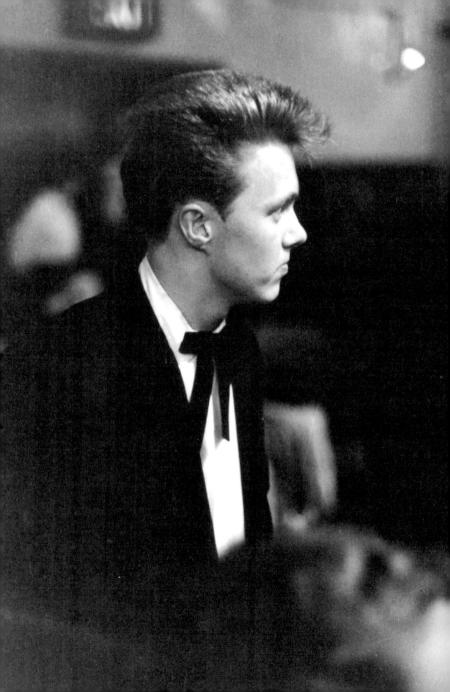

The Teddy Boys, or 'Teds', were the original teen rebels, the warning shot of generational turmoil in Britain following World War II. They set youth culture in motion, an early manifestation of working-class adolescent frustration and energy expressed through styling. The confrontational combination of old-fashioned clothing and racy rock 'n' roll hair is key to understanding the attitude and the look.

In the context of the class-conscious 1950s, the Teds' aim was to shock public decency and defy social conventions. Inspired by the elegant tailoring of the early 1900s (a style popular among upper-class young Guards officers), their neo-Edwardian style led the press to give them a common nickname for Edward: 'Teddy'.

But the Teddy Boys took this refined, formal look and subverted it, adding elements from popular Hollywood westerns in a mix of Pachuco and gun-slinger style. Rolled-up drainpipe trousers exposing brightly coloured socks; single-breasted, long-line and soft-fitting jackets with velvet lapels and cuffs; brocade waistcoats; narrow bow ties; and soft-soled, suede shoes known as brothel creepers (widely in use during World War II): the Teddy Boy look is truly a dandy's uniform. Minor variations and individual flourishes marked out the quality of the tailoring and state of the wearer's finances.

Before rock 'n' roll crossed the Atlantic and took the scene by storm, hitting the big screen in 1955 with MGM's scaremongering *Blackboard Jungle* (which featured the Bill Haley & His Comets hit 'Rock Around the Clock'), teenagers emulated the curls of actor Tony Curtis.

After Elvis, with many and reasonable variations according to skill and taste, male teens started to wear their hair longer, combed in a quiff — its most extreme version was large enough to warrant the name 'Elephant Trunk'. The sides were combed to the back to form the duck's arse. Needless to say, a great quantity of hair oil and brilliantine was needed to stabilize the hairstyle, and Brits used mainly Brylcreem. The original Teddy Boys' sideburns saw a resurgence in the 1970s, when they were worn very large and reaching the base of the earlobe.

THE TRUTH ABOUT
THE 'TEDDY BOYS'
AND THE TEDDY GIRLS

The 'Edwardians,' or 'Teddy Boys,' have been branded as hooligans, juvenile gangsters and delinquents. They have also been called dandies and mother's darlings. It is a confusing picture of exaggeration and distortion. A PICTURE POST *investigation seeks to bring it into focus. Our staff writer,* HILDE MARCHANT, *presents the facts. A* PSYCHIATRIST *of much experience with young people, interprets them.* JOSEPH McKEOWN *took the pictures*

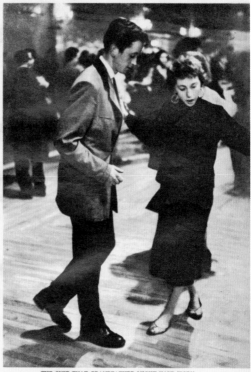

WE were in a dance-hall in Tottenham—a suburb of London—and the young men we wished to contact were distinctive and obvious. The floppy jackets hung to their knees, the poplin shirts were advertisement white, the trousers were ankle tight, the shoes were good black leather, and the ties were narrow bows. An ugly outfit? That is a matter of opinion; and we were not seeking opinion—only facts. To approach the facts meant we had first to approach the boys, talk to them, and challenge the honesty of their talk. And the first thing that struck me was that their clothes are deceptive. This Edwardian fashion gives a uniformity to a group of young people who are far from uniform. They are as varied, diverse and informal as any other group of human beings. They set a pattern in their velvet collars, dog-tooth checks and moccasin shoes. But there is no such standard pattern about their lives or behaviour.

But let them talk for themselves, for they are frank enough. What do they do during the day, or the week? One is a toy maker, one a glass cutter. Another is an engineer's apprentice, one a die cutter, another an electric welder and, surprisingly, another a National Serviceman on leave—back in his Teddy Boy civilian 'uniform.' (His hair was shorter than the others, but would still have horrified the Sergeant-major.) Their wages were good—ranging from the £4 17s. 6d. a week apprentice, to just over £12 a week for the skilled cabinet maker. Their suits cost between £17 and £20. All of them agreed that a good poplin shirt was just under £2 and that a pair of shoes was around the £3 mark. Most of them 'kept themselves'; which means they pay their parents something towards the rent and the household budget. Even so, pocket money was never less than £2 a week, and often double. They were not interested in drinks—a beer, perhaps, but more likely a mineral water. They

THE SUIT THAT GRANDFATHER MIGHT HAVE WORN
The dance is contemporary jive. But the suit is an adaptation of the Edwardian 'masher's' outfit. It is also English in conception and, unlike recent men's fashions, owes nothing to Hollywood.

25

Article published in *Picture Post* magazine, UK, 1954. *Previous spread*: A Teddy Boy at the Mecca Dance Hall in Tottenham, London, 1954

Do it yourself

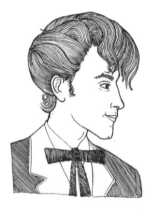

This version of the Teddy Boy haircut requires hair about twenty centimetres long on top

—

The top section is combed into a quiff falling towards the front, while the sides are tapered in order to be combed backwards to form a duck's arse

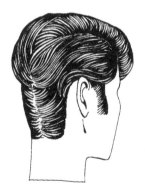

Hairspray can be used to stabilize the hairstyle

Total look

This style is all about confrontational contrasts: elegant Edwardian tailoring paired with overblown quiffs constructed with vast amounts of Brylcreem

The Edwardian drape jacket was adapted by rebellious British teens who took advantage of its numerous pockets to hide alcohol and other contraband

COMPLETE THE LOOK

with a single-breasted jacket with velvet lapels and cuffs, a fancy brocade waistcoat, slim drainpipe trousers and suede Gibson shoes. Top it off with a pair of bright socks and a narrow black bootlace bow

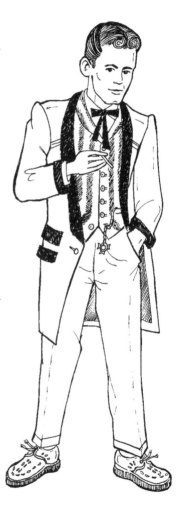

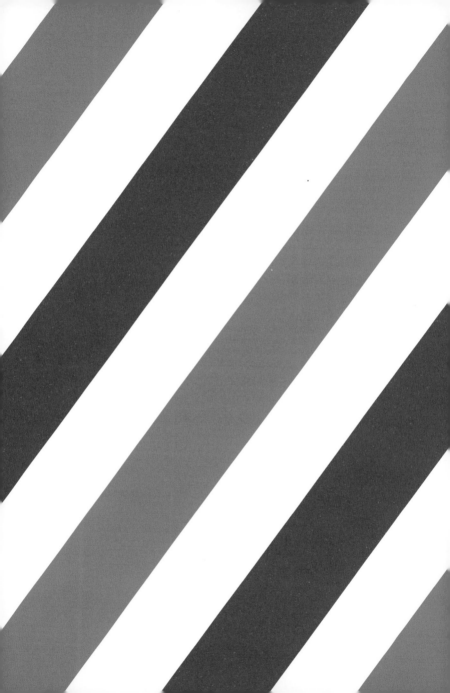

HIPSTER

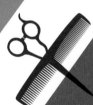

In the beginning, before Williamsburg, Shoreditch and artisan coffee, the clearest sign of the hipster's refusal of the American Way of Life was his hair. The post-war Beat Generation emulated the relaxed style and attitude of black musicians, repackaging an underground scene for alienated white youth. The Hipster haircut is a deliberate subversion of the uptight Crew Cut and the Ivy League, their clean lines grown untidily long and combed only with the hands.

The word 'hipster' came straight out of Harlem, from the African American jazz scene of the 1930s. It combines the adjective 'hip' or 'hep', meaning sophisticated and stylish, and the suffix '-ster' (like mobster, gangster). Being hip means being aware and in harmony with yourself. This philosophy appealed to the Beats, for whom *beat* might equally refer to a mystic beatific state or to being beaten down by the forces of materialism and conformism. Bewitched by the effortless cool of the musicians and the rhythm of bebop jazz, authors Jack Kerouac, Allen Ginsberg, Gregory Corso and Lawrence Ferlinghetti (who was the first to publish Ginsberg's generation-defining *Howl*, in 1956) projected the image of the hipster well beyond the cities of New York and San Francisco and into the global spotlight.

The hipster felt disconnected from the codes, morality and values of Western society following

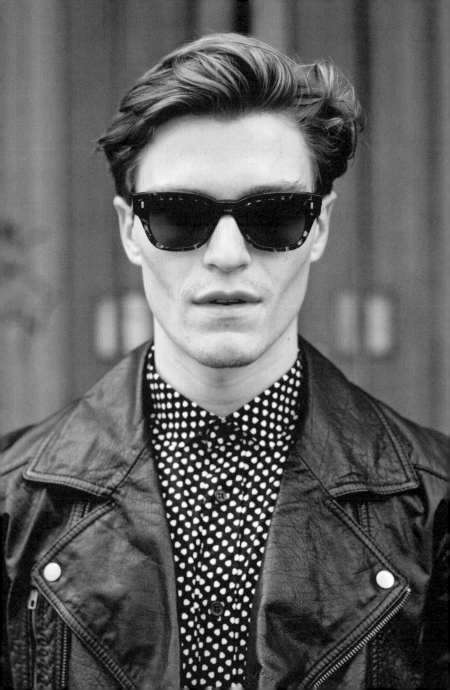

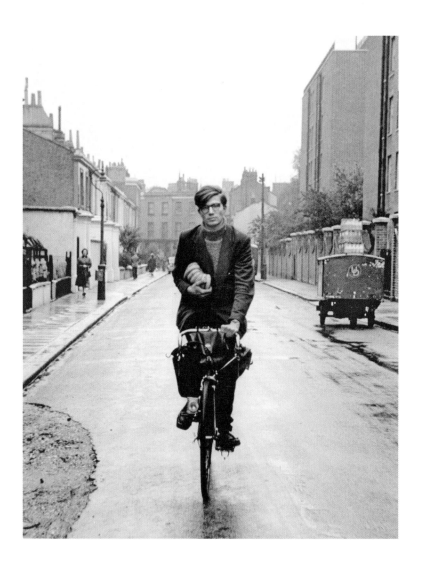

British author Colin Wilson riding his bike in Soho, London, 1956. *Previous spread:* A model sporting the classic 'just out of bed' modern hipster look

World War II. He identified with the poets, authors and artists of the Beat Generation set against the status quo of consumerism, militarism and puritanism advanced by the admen of Madison Avenue (see pp. 96–103). In his 1957 essay *The White Negro*, Norman Mailer paid homage to this new figure, describing him as a '*ménage-à-trois* between the bohemian, the juvenile delinquent and the Negro'. A fresh paradigm of masculinity, the hipster preferred the unexplored path of new experiences.

The hipster of 1950s' imagination could wander for months with no money in his pocket, sporting the scruffy and rundown look of the rough sleeper, without his charm being at all affected. He wore the second-hand clothes of factory workers and farmers (checked shirts, jeans, work jackets) and the louche, slouchy shapes of the jazz clubs (turtlenecks, sandals and sunglasses, even at night). Always out of shape and dishevelled, a hipster's hair looked as if he'd just got out of bed. The Hipster cut was a visible reminder that some things were beyond society's control.

Since the millennium, hipster style has seen a revival among young urbanites into retro and nerdy looks, consciously rejecting the mainstream. Its widespread appeal has been satirized in *The Hipster Handbook* (2003) and *HipsterMattic* (2011); the term itself is in increasingly pejorative use.

Do it yourself

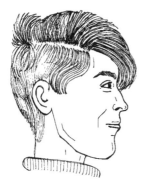

A longer variation of the well-groomed classics, the Crew Cut and Ivy League, this haircut requires medium long hair

—

At the sides, the hair is tapered. The top of the hair can be cut to various lengths, but is always visibly longer than the sides

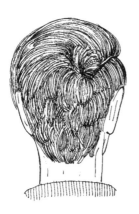

A parting — not necessarily straight — separates these sections. The hair is loosely styled, with no products

Total look

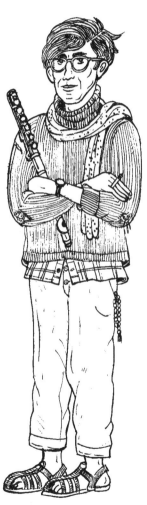

The original Hipsters of the Beat Generation rejected the values of consumerism and built their aesthetic on authenticity and self-expression

Today's Hipster is still opposed to mainstream fashion, but despite a nonchalant attitude, his style is far from accidental: every aspect of his look is carefully constructed

Visit your local second-hand shop for sartorial inspiration — avoid brands and labels and instead hunt out individual and one-off pieces

COMPLETE THE LOOK

with some vintage eyewear and a pair of brogues with no socks

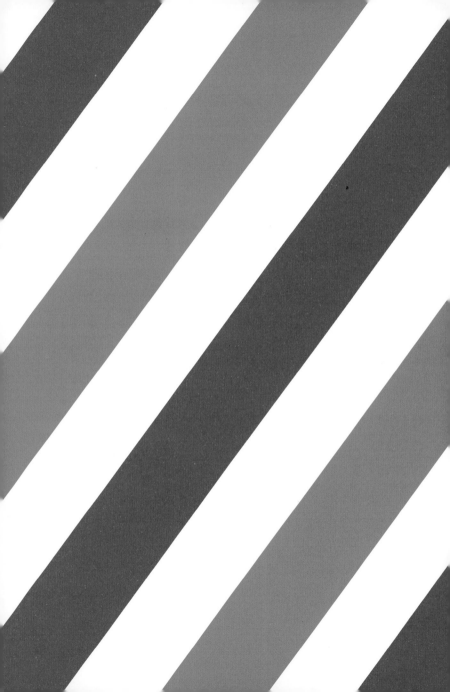

UNTAMED BEARD

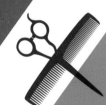

The Untamed Beard conjures up a romantic image of revolutionaries and folk heroes. Giuseppe Garibaldi led his one thousand men, largely volunteers, into battle in 1860 dressed in their own crumpled shirts, with unkempt hair and long beards, and took Sicily. A century later, Fidel Castro's scruffy partisan rebels overthrew Fulgencio Batista (a Slick Back man), freeing Cuba from US imperialism. These fighters vowed to cut neither their hair nor beards until the revolution had been achieved, and were given the nickname *Los Barbudos* (The Bearded Ones).

Stalked by Batista's army, the *Barbudos* continued the guerrilla war for three years (1956–9) in the wild forests of the Sierra Maestra, their beards providing protection against the cold, the heat and the sun. The Untamed Beard was also an effective identifying mark of membership that helped them to spot infiltrators: a source of pride, its extent signalled length of service. Once the local people, the reporters and the press became familiar with these revolutionaries, their beards came to symbolize the revolution against a corrupt authoritarian regime.

Despite, or perhaps because of, strong opposition from the United States government, these rebels captured the imagination of disaffected American youths, to whom Cuba exemplified idealistic socialist politics. The failed attempt to overthrow Castro's new

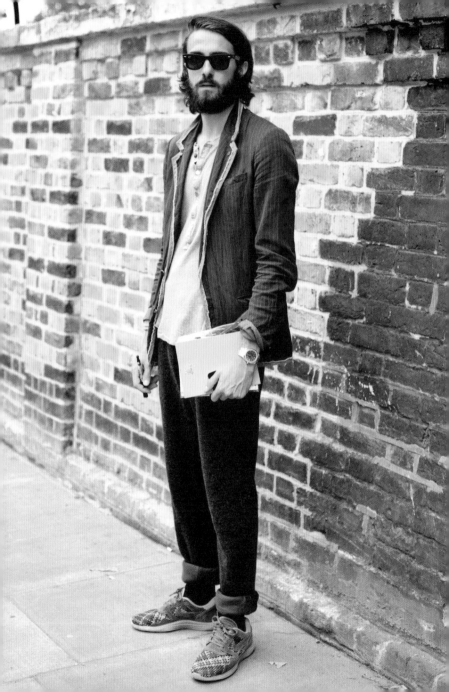

government during the Bay of Pigs invasion in 1961 only increased their appeal. Argentinian fighter–philosopher Che Guevara, Castro's brother-in-arms, brought glamour to Marxism, captured in iconic photographs by Alberto Korda and Magnum staffer René Burri. Even today this revolutionary with the Untamed Beard is a pin-up on student walls the world over.

In recent years the beard in all its endless variety has reached near-ubiquity among fashionable men. The Untamed Beard remains the mark of the outsider, of opposition — its signal is the call of the wild man, the call to revolution.

Cuban revolutionary Camilo Cienfuegos after the invasion of Cuba, 1959
Previous spread: Model sporting the contemporary urban beard look

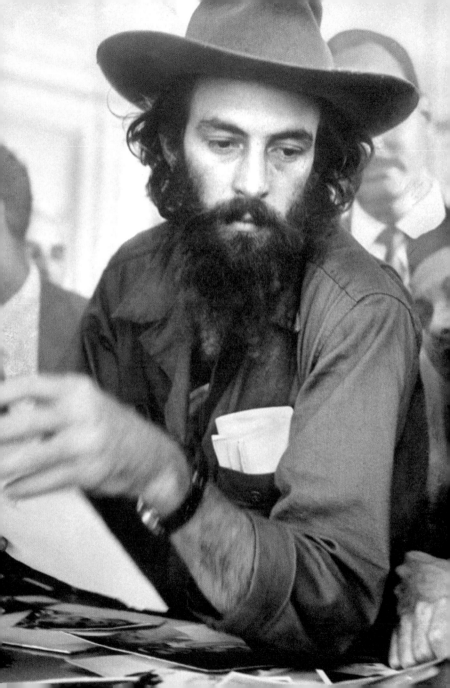

Do it yourself

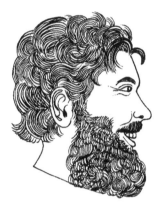

Starting from a long haircut, this style does not need any particular treatment

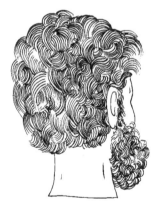

The beard is left ungroomed, with no razor regulation

Total look

Traditionally, thick, ungroomed beards and long hair protected their bearers from extreme weather

Today, a more groomed look is preferred, adapting this wild style for a more urban environment

COMPLETE THE LOOK

with a large plaid shirt buttoned to the top, leather braces, dark denim jeans and leather boots

This style works particularly well when paired with a hat: whether Che Guevara's iconic black beret, Camilo Cienfuegos's signature Stetson or the standard military Ridgeway Cap

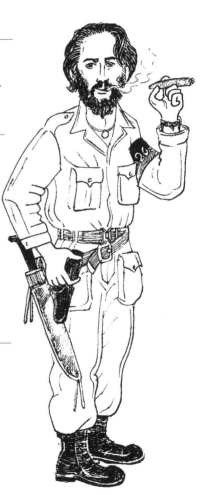

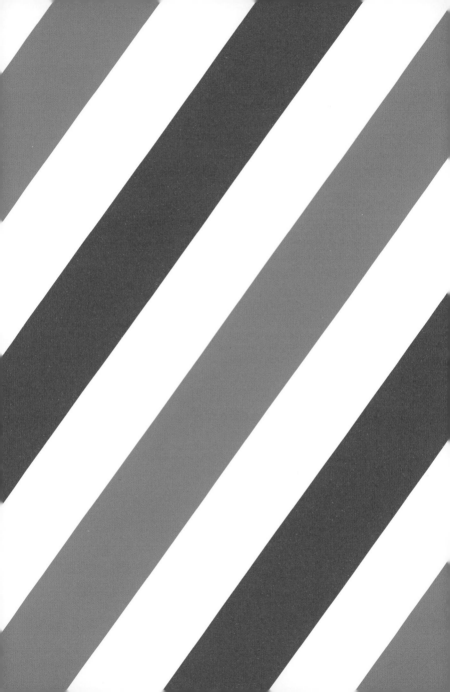

MOD

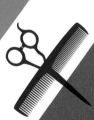

Neat, clean and sharp — three adjectives that define the Mod look — clash with the image of post-war Britain as a land of rationing and rubble. Yet, at the turn of the 1960s a group of men saw a self-determined future better than their parents' and ran towards it. Youths not yet into their twenties decided that the world was theirs, that it was modern, and that they would embody its values, in fashion and hairstyles.

Years of austerity followed World War II. The Mods came of age in a Britain beginning to recover, but before London began to swing. A newly formed welfare state and the seeds of prosperity gave the working-class teens of Pimlico and Belgravia a pay cheque that allowed them to prove that a three-button made-to-measure suit was the best social leveller. Against the old Britain of hand-me-downs, smoky pubs and warm beers, the Mods proposed coffee shops and sartorial precision — all things new, smart, ultramodern and cool. Their outlook was international, while uniquely British: the sleek design of Vespa and Lambretta scooters replaced the rattling BSA Bantam, and Tony Curtis's wild and sweaty rock 'n' roll was snubbed in favour of R&B and soul music sounds. Tight jeans, stripy button-down shirts and Italian-style short jackets were all the rage; hair was short, but had flair.

Haircuts were key in the carefully polished Mod image. To have a properly executed Perry Como

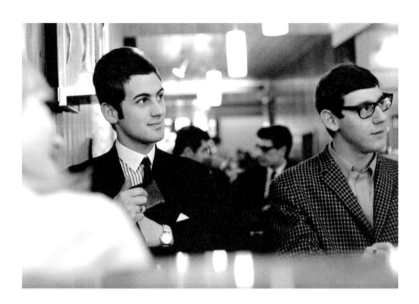

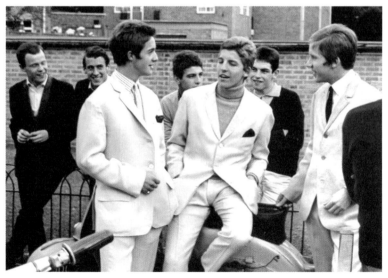

How to Cut the New French Line

THIS is a classic interpretation of the new Club line for men, launched by the French men's hairdressing *Syndicat*. It is quiet and sober in its design but smart and groomed enough for any age group.

The hair is a little longer than in most recent men's lines. It is not so much thinned by the razor as carefully refined.

Fig. 1.– After having put in the parting (1) make a division through the hair just above the temple (A).

By making a second division a little lower (B), one can shield the "shoulder" meshes which correspond to the area of the greatest volume in the finished style.

The base of the sides is thinned vertically according to the shape of the head.

Fig. 2.– The back and nape hair is reduced with the razor, the scissors being used to control only the extreme points.

All the overlapping meshes on the top of the head must be gone over again very lightly with the razor to obtain a good blending of the points, while retaining fullness just below the parting.

Fig. 3.– In dressing out, secure volume at the sides by taking a small round styling brush and, having determined the thickness of the mesh (1) place the brush at the root (2). Lift the hair with a turning movement while directing the hot air jet from the dryer on to top of the hair (3).

Fig. 4.– To obtain a natural volume at the level of the parting, force the roots a little with the comb *against* the natural direction of the hair growth.

Except for smoothing the hair, take care not to flatten the volume which has been achieved.

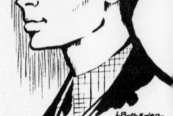

by

Fernand Gautier

Member of the Syndicat de la Haute Coiffure Masculine and of the Comité Artistique de la Coiffure Française

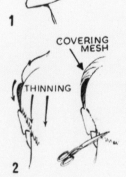

COVERING MESH

THINNING

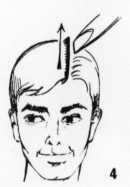

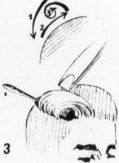

or French Crop was no simple task. The barber's tribulations started when he was asked for a 'no-product haircut', meaning a cut that required no use of brilliantine. This was a great innovation in men's hair fashion. The Mods shunned the scarcely hygienic hair pomades and oils, opting instead for haircuts with a shape defined by razor and tapering.

After running battles between Mods and the slightly older Rockers took place along the seafront from Brighton to Margate in 1964, being Mod fell out of favour. Its most visible contemporary ambassadors were The Who; revivalists include the 'Modfather' Paul Weller in the late 1970s, and Mod hair enthusiasts Oasis during the 1990s.

Hairdressers' Journal, 1963. *Previous spread:* Young and smartly dressed British Mods, London, 1960s

Do it yourself

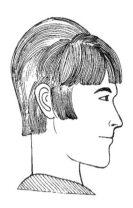

The Mods' 'New French Line' has a short fringe cut about three centimetres above the eyebrows

—

Hair can be of different lengths, falling in its natural position

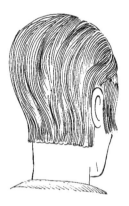

Sideburns reach the ear lobe, while the nape of the neck is left full, usually with an uneven edge

—

The upper back section is backcombed, or 'teased', and fixed with hairspray

Total look

First sported by teenagers in London at the turn of the 1960s, this polished look is inspired by Italian style yet remains uniquely British

The innovative tapered shape of this cut means that no styling products are required

COMPLETE THE LOOK

with a roll-neck jumper and short Italian jacket, drainpipe jeans and winklepicker shoes. Top it off with an oversized military parka

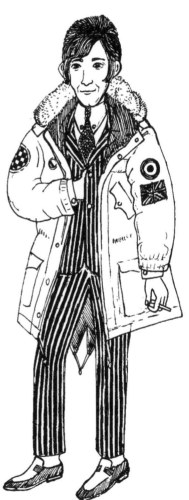

MOP TOP

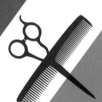

When The Beatles landed in New York in 1964 for their first US tour, they took the country by storm. Paul McCartney is on record as attributing this in part to their iconic hairstyle. Despite some scathing reviews — 'four British lads who sing when they are not busy running away from barbers' read the Associated Press report — the impact of the lovable Mop Tops was immediate.

In a nation where the Crew Cut was the male haircut par excellence, teenagers were fascinated by The Beatles' look, and the usual 'short back and sides' was soon forgotten. Barber shops were deserted: The Beatles — and their hair — became a matter of public importance. In the context of the pop avant-garde, the Mop Top was regarded as a sign of modernity rather than necessarily of rebellion. A hairstyle that didn't require hair pomades or brilliantine, it was part of a new conception of men's fashion, which was also apparent in the Mods' New French Line. Long cuts and natural styling for men were gaining global acceptance.

They owe it all to sex and Hamburg. The Beatles used to wear Rockabilly quiffs and DAs ('duck's arses') like most Western young people in the late 1950s. The great change happened after a spate of performances in the German city in 1960, and thanks to the intervention of two key figures in the history of the

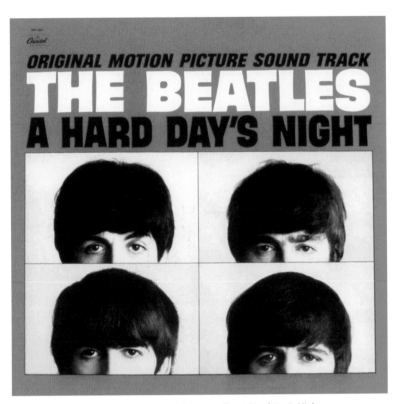

The Mop Top was the main protagonist of the 1964 film *A Hard Day's Night*

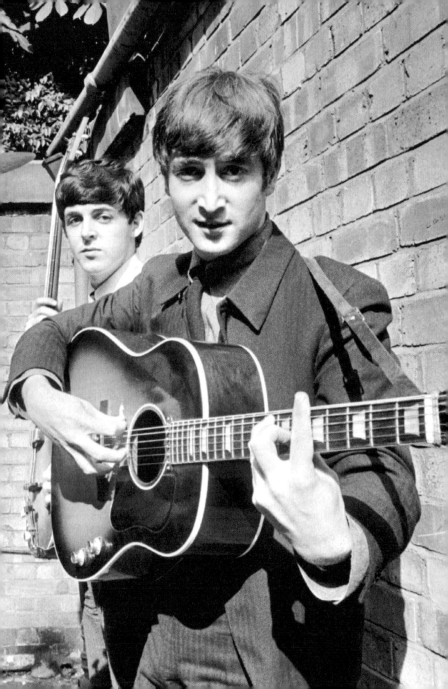

band: Astrid Kirchherr, a student at the local fashion academy (now a photographer), and Stuart Sutcliffe, the fifth member of the group (who died prematurely in 1962). Stuart fell in love with Astrid and, under her careful guidance, was the first Beatle to ditch the Brylcreem and leave his forelock to fall freely on his forehead. Similar haircuts were common in Hamburg among the Beatniks and the Exies, the German existentialists: in Germany the cut was known as der Pilzkopf (the Mushroom Head). At first, the band was amused by the cut, but soon John, Paul and George decided to follow Stuart's example. Only Pete, the drummer in the group's early days, did not embrace the look. History has it that shortly after, he was asked to leave the band and Ringo took his place.

Paul McCartney and John Lennon, London, 1963

Do it yourself

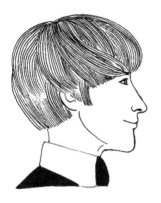

A long haircut, with the top part of the hair brought forwards and combed to the side

—

The back and sides need very little tapering and layering to convey a natural effect and increase volume

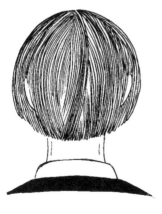

The hairstyle does not require any product, though a little bit of hairspray will keep the forelock to the side

Total look

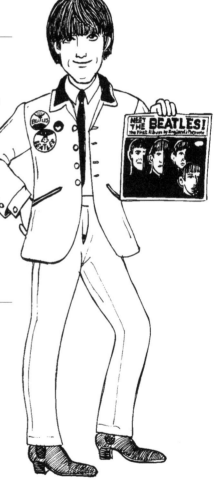

The Mop Top look was pioneered by The Beatles' long shaggy haircut with floppy fringe, so it's no surprise that the total look is inspired by the iconic pop group

The four Brits still inspire fashion today: John Lennon's signature round glasses and T-shirts with The Beatles prints are a must-have for every nostalgic rock fan

COMPLETE THE LOOK

with a collarless jacket or blazer over a white shirt with a pair of Cuban heeled, tight fitting ankle-length 'Beatle boots'

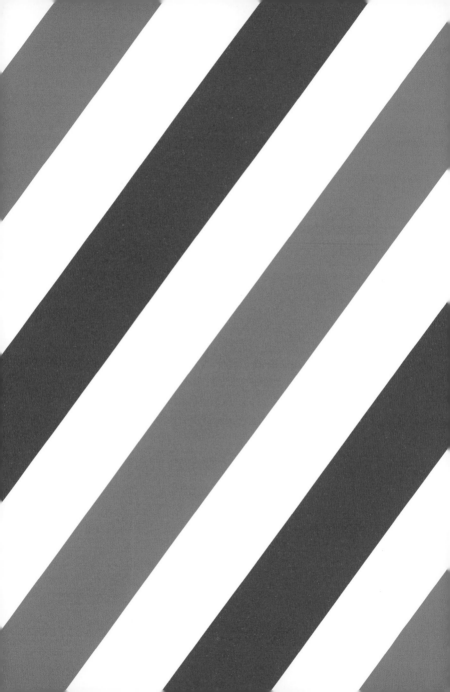

AFRO

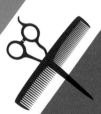

The Afro celebrates the natural beauty of curly hair, particularly the tightly coiled and textured, 'nappy' hair of Black Africans. Hair is encouraged to follow its natural growth pattern in a voluminous halo effect around the head. Wearing an Afro was once a political statement of identity and empowerment; today it's about fashion.

In the late nineteenth century, African Americans, Afro-Caribbeans and other black peoples began to use heavy cosmetics to style their hair, weighing down their curls in an attempt to adhere to Caucasian standards of beauty. The hair industry's response was to develop a wide range of products to enable this assimilation, ranging from mechanical hair straighteners and hot combs to chemical hair relaxers and hair weaves (which attach Caucasian hair extensions to the hair root). The market today is worth billions of dollars.

Undergoing these laborious and sometimes damaging or painful hair treatments was an everyday routine for both men and women until the mid-1960s, when the US Civil Rights Movement succeeded in getting new equal-rights legislation passed. A new black awareness arose promoting ethnic diversity and identity as valuable rather than a mark of shame to be hidden. The revolutionary Black Panthers chanted the motto 'Black is Beautiful'; an Afro-wearing James

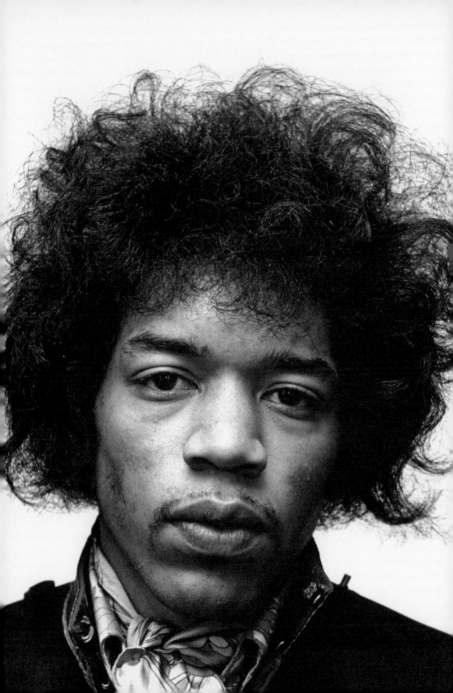

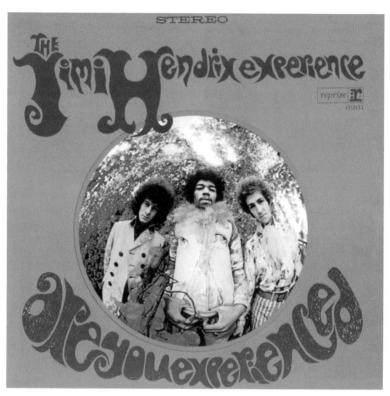

American edition of the *Are You Experienced* album by The Jimi Hendrix Experience group, 1967. *Previous page:* Jimi Hendrix, 1967

Brown released 'Say It Loud, I'm Black And I'm Proud', echoing the words of Martin Luther King, in 1968. The Afro became one of the major emblems of 1960s' counterculture.

The growing success of black music played a crucial role in the rise in popularity of the Afro hairstyle. At the time of his debut with the Isley Brothers (1964–5), even Jimi Hendrix was straightening his hair. His transformation — to Afroed musical superstar — came in London. During the tour of his debut 1966 album *Are You Experienced* the other two (white) members of the band joined Jimi's 'hair performance' and stepped on stage with backcombed, or 'teased', Afros of their own. The following year the musical *Hair* debuted off-Broadway, presenting a new and exciting androgynous figure — free, happy and surrounded by a halo of picked-out curly hair — to a mainstream audience.

Hairstyles became a novel pathway to racial integration. When the Afro style reached Africa in the mid-1970s, the social elite embraced it, wearing it as a sign of modernity and a more Western and progressive look. It came full circle in Tanzania, where it was prohibited as a form of cultural neo-colonization.

Do it yourself

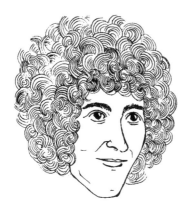

Hair is cut medium to long all over the head, following the roundness of the skull, and left to stand away from the root

—

If hair is not naturally curly, backcombing, or 'teasing', can deliver a similar effect

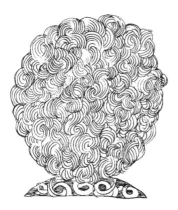

African hair often requires no product; Caucasian hair may require gels or hairspray to maintain volume

Total look

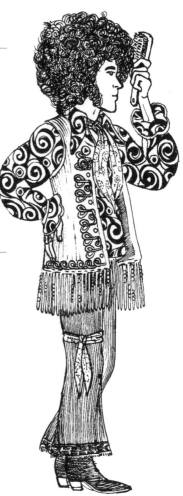

The flamboyant Afro is a clear statement of pride and self-acceptance

Create a splendid 1970s disco outfit by pairing bell-bottom trousers with a loose-fitting and colourful Dashiki shirt

COMPLETE THE LOOK

with bright colours and frantic patterns plus a range of fanciful accessories, such as a coloured headband, retro round sunglasses and big bracelets

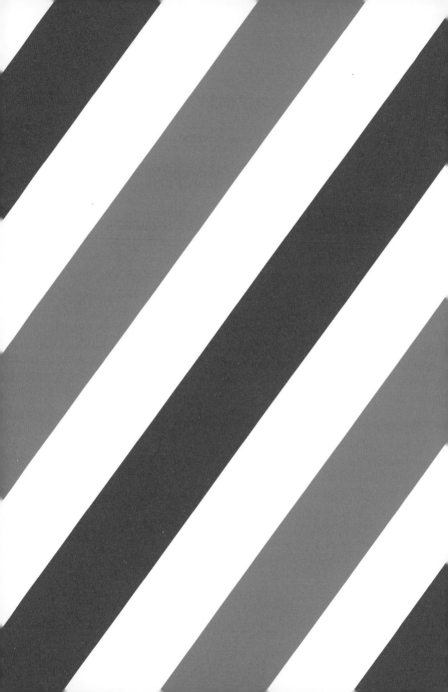

SKINHEAD

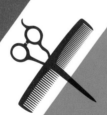

At the end of the 1970s, the New Agers' hopes for a new world, an Age of Aquarius based on 'harmony and understanding … mystic crystal revelations', racial and gender equality, was fading after a decade. In fact, there were some people among the British working class whose views directly opposed those ideals, and a group had begun forming since the 1960s. Hair was used to carry these messages — on the one side there was the Afro and the loose, long hair of the counterculture, and on the other, the Skinheads.

A hard-core version of the Mods, the Skins saw themselves as defending British values from the threat of widespread consumerism by holding up old-fashioned, patriotic working-class pride against middle-class hedonism. In their view, Hippies, Pakistanis and homosexuals were visible proof of British society's imminent collapse. These groups were the targets of the first Skinhead attacks that garnered widespread media attention in 1969–70. Although this kind of class war did not admit any vandalism or robbery, violence surely played a role.

The Skinheads were a pseudo-militia, ready to defend their nation. The defining characteristic of their uniform was a shaved head, which earned them several other nicknames: peanuts, lemons, cropheads, boiled eggs and skulls. The one they chose, that stuck,

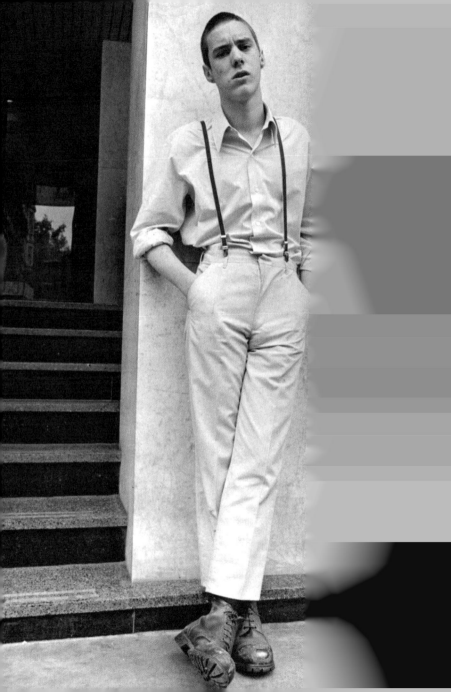

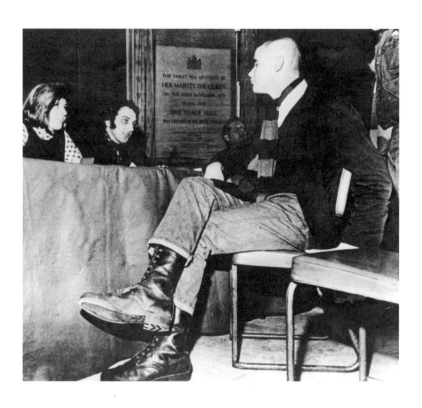

Skinhead in London, 1970. *Previous spread:* A Skinhead wearing slacks with braces, London, 1969

took on aggressive overtones. Short, skinny trousers, rolled-up jeans, military bomber jackets, crisp white or checked button-down shirts, braces and combat boots (sometimes with a steel toe) exaggerated the hypermasculine image of pure proletarian force, where no frills or embellishments were admitted. To perfect the Skinhead look, the most minimal of minimalist haircuts had the biggest impact: the shaved head was a clear symbol of military rigour, hygiene and levelling. The perfect uniformity of their heads all in line tolerated no compromise. Hair was cut with electric clippers or, during the 1980s, with open razor blades, to a length ranging from one to four millimetres.

Although a first phase ended in the early 1970s, a new breed of Skinheads emerged a decade later, bringing with them the overt violence of the far right wing. The style spread to Australia, the United States and Europe, particularly Germany. Links with neo-Nazism were explored in the 1992 film *Romper Stomper*. 'Skinhead' became a synonym for racism and oppression, far removed from the Jamaican roots of the ska and reggae rhythms pumping in the veins of this subculture during its early days, when members stormed the dance floor at gigs by Madness and The Specials. At a time of no jobs, no money, the anger of the Sex Pistols' 'No Future', Skinheads turned to the nihilism of Punk.

Do it yourself

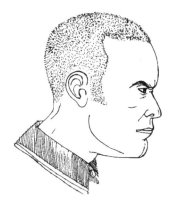

Hair is cut with a razor, or clippers set at one to four millimetres

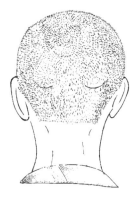

In its longest version, hair up to five millimetres, a side parting can be shaved with a razor to give more shape to the cut

Total look

This hypermasculine cut was originally a reaction against mainstream values

Perfect for the late riser with a rebellious attitude, the Skinhead look requires minimal styling

COMPLETE THE LOOK

with a band T-shirt, rolled-up or cut-off drainpipe jeans, a pair of Dr. Marten's boots and an impressive set of tattoos

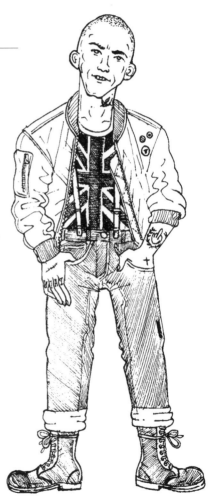

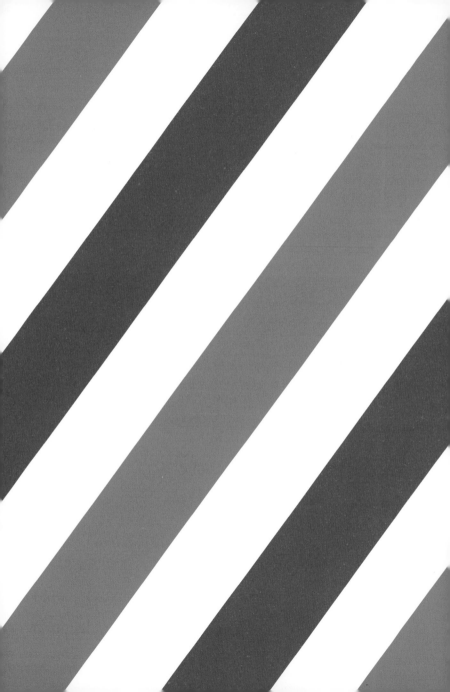

ARTIST

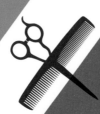

Declaring yourself an artist perhaps gives you licence to greater sartorial freedom. Hair is no exception. Unusual clothes and accessories, and wild hairstyles in particular characterized many twentieth-century artists from Salavador Dalí and his flamboyant moustache to Andy Warhol in a lopsided wig.

It should be no surprise that many of the most inventive hairstyles asked of a barber today were first tested, sometimes decades ago, on the heads of creative types and intellectuals. This phenomenon was especially visible among the French avant-garde. It was in Paris that the first upright hair, the first crazy haircuts, the first hair dyes and application of organic substances to the hair made their public appearance.

The craze began with the *poètes maudits* (literally, 'accursed poets' — but any artist or writer living outside societal rules) and a myth about Baudelaire's green hair, which was probably a scalp preparation to treat baldness. But it was the Surrealists who made hair truly a field of psychological and symbolic analysis, and their abundant production of works dedicated to hair is there to prove it.

Paintings and sculptures were not enough to satisfy the Surrealists' desire to astound and experiment, and so their own heads came into play, serving

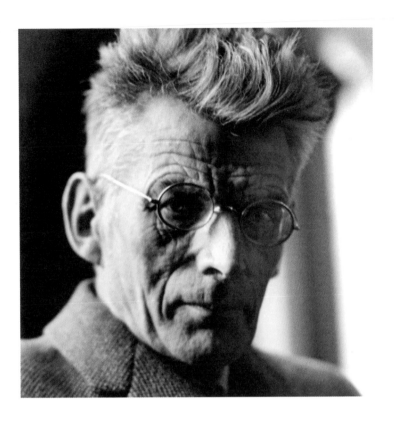

Irish novelist and playwright Samuel Beckett, 1960s

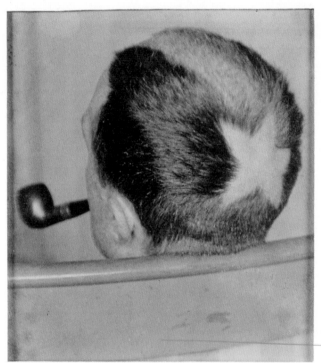

Tonsure (Paris, 1919), a photograph of Dadaist artist Marcel Duchamp's head

a creative flair that was in no need of any recognition from the world of fashion. After all, one of their goals was to condemn the bourgeois lifestyle, and what could possibly be more provocative than a disquieting and crazy everyday look?

Marcel Duchamp's *Tonsure* (1921) is a star shape razored into the back of his hair by George de Zayas, indicating that the place for art is in (or on) the head; Yves Tanguy wore a gravity-defying quiff; Jean Cocteau explosive curls. The sheer force of Irish playwright, director and poet Samuel Beckett's intellect seemed to push the hair out through the top of his head into a bristly, gravity-defying hairstyle, making him instantly recognizable and adding to his fame. It is worth noting that he, too, lived most of his adult life in Paris.

Do it yourself

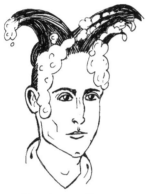

MARCEL DUCHAMP

Artists' haircuts do not follow any instructions: that is the point. They are instead pure individualistic experimentation

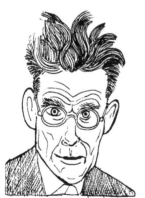

SAMUEL BECKETT

Techniques and tools serve to allow free expression of body and soul, even if the tools involved are the most traditional ones, such as the razor, employed to create cut-out patterns, or soap, used as a precursor to hair gel

Total look

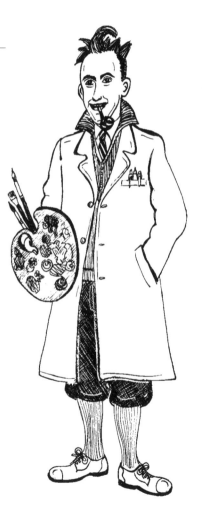

This look is undefined, original, creative and nonconformist. Treat your hair as a blank canvas — your head is just another art medium

COMPLETE THE LOOK

however you wish: there are no rules. Standards of good taste and mainstream fashion trends don't apply to you

You can always go for the art student look: paint-splattered dungarees, mismatched socks, facial piercings and dark circles under the eyes

Inspired? Check out our A–Z of some of the world's trendiest barber shops...

AUSTRALIA

PICKINGS & PARRY
126 Gertrude Street, Fitzroy
Melbourne, Victoria 3065
+61 394173390
www.pickingsandparry.com
Opening hours .... Open 7 days
Booking .... Telephone

SAMUEL J FORDYCE BARBER SHOP
Captains of Industry
2 Somerset Place
Melbourne, Victoria 3000
+61 396704405
www.captainsofindustry.com.au
Opening hours .. Closed Monday & Sunday
Booking .... Online and telephone

UNCLE JOE'S BARBER SHOP
74–76 King Street
Perth, Western Australia 6000
+61 417783222
www.unclejoes.com.au
Opening hours .... Closed Sunday
Booking .... Online and telephone

WESTONS BARBERSHOP
456 William Street
Perth, Western Australia 6000
+61 892282692
www.westonsbarbers.com
Opening hours .... Closed Sunday
Booking .... Telephone

THE BARBER SHOP
89 York Street
Central Business District
Sydney, New South Wales 2000
+61 292999699
www.thisisthebarbershop.com
Opening hours .... Closed Sunday
Booking .... Telephone

THE HAPPY SAILORS BARBERSHOP
748 Bourke Street
Redfern
Sydney, New South Wales 2016
+61 296901452
www.thehappysailorsbarbershop.com.au
Opening hours .... Closed Sunday
Booking .... Telephone and email

CLEVELAND'S SALON & CAFÉ
311 Cleveland Street
Redfern
Sydney, New South Wales 2016
+61 296988449
www.clevelandsoncleveland.com
Opening hours .... Open 7 days
Booking .... Telephone

AUSTRIA

BROTHER'S BARBERSHOP
Neubaugasse 81
Vienna 1070
+43 19908304
www.barbershop.wien
Opening hours .. Closed Monday & Sunday
Booking .... Online and telephone

CANADA

ATELIER FRANK & OAK BARBERS
160 Rue Saint Viateur Est 105
Montreal, QC, H2T 1A8
+1 5142281366
www.frankandoak.com/atelier
Opening hours .. Closed Tuesday & Sunday
Booking .... Online

VICTORY BARBER & BRAND
1315 Blanshard Street
Victoria, BC, V8V 0B5
+1 2503811522
www.victorybarbers.com
Opening hours .... Open 7 days
Booking .... Telephone

DIRECTORY

DENMARK

CARL'S BARBER SHOP
Østerbrogade 43, Østerbro
Copenhagen 2100
+45 26782222
www.carlsbarbershop.dk
Opening hours .... Closed Sunday
Booking .... Online

FRANCE

LA BOUCHERIE
36 Cours Evrard de Fayolle
Bordeaux 33000
+33 557295120
Opening hours .. Closed Monday & Sunday
Booking .... Telephone and email

LES MAUVAIS GARÇONS
Le Bon Marché Rive Gauche
24 Rue de Sèvres
Paris 75007
+33 142223419
www.lesmauvaisgarcons.fr
Opening hours .... Closed Sunday
Booking .... Telephone

GERMANY

BARBERSHOP COLOGNE
Brüsseler Strasse 90
50672 Cologne
+49 22194529000
www.barbershop-cologne.de
Opening hours .. Closed Monday & Sunday
Booking .... Telephone and email

TORRETO BARBERSHOP
Alte Gasse 38
60313 Frankfurt am Main
+49 6926090261
www.torreto-barbershop.de
Opening hours .. Closed Monday & Sunday
Booking .... Telephone

GREECE

1900 THE BARBER SHOP
Ypsilandou 35 & Ploutarchou - Kolonaki
Athens 106 76
+30 2107220511
Opening hours .... Closed Sunday
Booking .... Telephone

IRELAND

THE DEMON BARBERS
The Ink Factory
15 Wellington Quay
Dublin 2, County Dublin
+353 16708641
www.theinkfactory.ie/demon-barbers
Opening hours .... Open 7 days
Booking .... Telephone and walk in

GROOMING ROOMS
16 South William Street
Dublin 2, County Dublin
+353 16790777
www.thegroomingrooms.com
Opening hours .... Closed Sunday
Booking .... Online and telephone

ITALY

BULLFROG
Via Dante 4
Milan 20121
+39 289096163
www.bullfrogbarbershop.com
Opening hours .. Closed Monday & Sunday
Booking .... Telephone and email

TONSOR CLUB
Via Palermo 15
Milan 20121
+39 249533040
www.tonsorclub.com
Opening hours .. Closed Monday & Sunday
Booking ...... Online, telephone and email

NETHERLANDS

BARBER
Binnen Oranjestraat 24
Amsterdam 1013 JA
+31 203373755
www.barber.nl
Opening hours .. Closed Monday & Sunday
Booking .... Online

HUTSPOT
Van Woustraat 4
Amsterdam 1073 LL
+31 202231331
www.hutspotamsterdam.com
Opening hours .... Closed Monday
Booking .... Online and telephone

NEW YORK BARBERSHOP
Hotel New York
Koninginnenhoofd 1
Rotterdam 3072 AD
+31 104853196
www.newyorkbarbershop.nl
Opening hours .. Closed Monday & Sunday
Booking .... Telephone

SCHOREM BARBIER
Nieuwe Binnenweg 104
Rotterdam 3015 BD
+31 102410309
www.schorembarbier.nl
Opening hours .. Closed Monday & Sunday
Booking .... No bookings

NEW ZEALAND

MALONEY'S BARBER SHOP
1–192 Victoria Street West
Auckland City
Auckland 1010
+64 93793060
www.maloneys.co.nz
Opening hours .... Closed Sunday
Booking .... No booking except for shaves

PORTUGAL

FIGAROS BARBERSHOP
Rua do Alecrim 39, Chiado
Lisbon 1200-014
+ 351 213470199
www.figaroslisboa.com
Opening hours .. Closed Monday & Sunday
Booking .... No bookings

O PURISTA BARBIERE
Rua Nova da Trindade 16C, Chiado
Lisbon 1200-303
+351 916442744
Opening hours .... Closed Monday
Booking .... Telephone and Facebook

RUSSIA

BOY CUT
14/8 Bersenevskaya naberezhnaya
Moscow 119072
+7 4955184909
www.boycut.ru
Opening hours .... Open 7 days
Booking .... Telephone

CHOP-CHOP
9/3 Stoleshnikov Lane
Moscow 125009
+7 4951500282
www.chopchop.me
Opening hours .... Open 7 days
Booking .... Online and telephone

SPAIN

ONE O NINE
Carrer Mare de Déu Del Pilar 15
Barcelona 08003
+34 930016992
109.es
Opening hours .. Closed Monday & Sunday
Booking .... Telephone and email

DIRECTORY

ÁLVARO THE BARBER
Calle Gonzalo de Berceo 46
Logroño 26005
+34 941202149
Opening hours .... Closed Sunday
Booking .... Telephone and email

MALAYERBA
Plaza Dos de Mayo 3
Madrid 28004
+34 912163900
www.barberiamalayerba.es
Opening hours .. Closed Monday & Sunday
Booking .... Telephone and email

SWEDEN

SHARPER OF SWEDEN
Prinsgatan 6
Gothenburg 41305
+46 31240506
www.sharperbarbershop.se
Opening hours .. Closed Monday & Sunday
Booking .... Online and telephone

BARBER & BOOKS
Östgötagatan 21
Stockholm 11625
+46 86400227
www.barberandbooks.se
Opening hours .... Closed weekends
Booking .... Online and telephone

SWITZERLAND

AVEDA BARBERSHOP
Alfred-Escherstrasse 23
Zurich 8002
+41 433171131
www.eddine.ch
Opening hours .. Closed Monday & Sunday
Booking .... Online and telephone

UNITED KINGDOM

THE DERRY BARBER COMPANY
22 Great James Street
Derry BT48 7DA, Northern Ireland
+44 2871261067
www.thederrybarbercompany.com
Opening hours .... Closed Sunday
Booking .... Telephone

RUFFIANS
23 Queensferry Street
Edinburgh EH2 4QS, Scotland
+44 1312258962
www.ruffians.co.uk
Opening hours .... Closed Sunday
Booking .... Telephone and email

THE LOFT BARBERS LOUNGE
1 Okehampton Street
Exeter EX4 1DW, England
+44 1392257400
www.theloftbarbers.com
Opening hours .... Closed Sunday
Booking .... Telephone and email

PRIMO GENTLEMENS BARBER
18 Wilson Street, The Merchant City
Glasgow G1 1SS, Scotland
+44 1415528793
primobarber.tumblr.com
Opening hours .... Open 7 days
Booking .... No bookings

BARBER BARBER
Barton Arcade, 3 Deansgate
Manchester M3 2BH, England
+44 1618325409
www.barberbarber.net
Opening hours .... Open 7 days
Booking .... Telephone

DIRECTORY

THE BOX & BARBER CAFÉ
3–5 Bank street
Newquay TR7 1EP, England
+44 7590008007
Opening hours .... Closed Sunday
Booking .... Telephone

SCRAGG'S BARBERSHOP
91A-93 Lark Lane
Liverpool L17 8UP, England
+44 7890109223
www.scraggsbarbershop.com
Opening hours .... Closed Sunday
Booking .... Telephone

BARBER & PARLOUR
64–66 Redchurch Street
London E2 7DP, England
+44 2033761777
www.barberandparlour.com
Opening hours .... Open 7 days
Booking .... Online and telephone

CARTER AND BOND
Woodhouse
189 Westbourne Grove
London W11 2SB, England
+44 2089620484
www.carterandbond.com
Opening hours .. Closed Monday & Sunday
Booking .... Telephone

DOLCE & GABBANA BARBERSHOP
53–55 New Bond Street
London W1S 1DG, England
+44 2074959250
www.dolcegabbana.com
Opening hours .... Open 7 days
Booking .... Telephone

GENTLEMEN'S TONIC
31A Bruton Place
London W1J 6NN, England
+44 2072974343
www.gentlemenstonic.com
Opening hours .... Open 7 days
Booking .... Online

GEO F TRUMPER
9 Curzon Street
London W1J 5HQ, England
+44 2074991850
www.trumpers.com
Opening hours .... Closed Sunday
Booking .... Telephone

HUCKLE THE BARBER
340 Old Street
London EC1V 9DS, England
+44 2032220021
www.hucklethebarber.com
Opening hours .... Closed Sunday
Booking .... Online and telephone

JOE AND CO
22 Peter Street
London W1F 0AG, England
+44 2077347000
www.joeandco.net
Opening hours .. Closed Monday & Sunday
Booking .... Online and telephone

MURDOCK AT LIBERTY
210–220 Regent Street
London W1B 5AH, England
+44 2033937946
www.murdocklondon.com
Opening hours .... Open 7 days
Booking .... Telephone

PALL MALL BARBERS
27 Whitcomb Street
London WC2H 7EP, England
+44 2079307787
www.pallmallbarbers.com
Opening hours .... Closed Sunday
Booking .... Online and telephone

PANKHURST
10 Newburgh Street
London W1F 7RN, England
+44 2072879955
www.pankhurstlondon.com
Opening hours .... Open 7 days
Booking .... Telephone

DIRECTORY

RUFFIANS
27 Maiden Lane
London WC2E 7JS, England
+44 2072408180
www.ruffians.co.uk
Opening hours .... Open 7 days
Booking .... Telephone and email

SHARPS BARBER AND SHOP
9 Windmill Street
London W1T 2JF, England
+44 2076368688
www.sharpsbarbers.com
Opening hours .... Open 7 days
Booking .... Telephone

TED'S OTTOMAN LOUNGE
31 Theobalds Road
London WC1X 8SP, England
+44 2078316463
www.tedsgroomingroom.com
Opening hours .... Open 7 days
Booking .... Online and telephone

THE BARBER AT ALFRED DUNHILL
2 Davies Street
London W1K 3DJ, England
+44 2078534440
www.dunhill.com/en/London
Opening hours .... Closed Sunday
Booking .... Online and telephone

THE REFINERY
60 Brook Street
London W1K 5DU, England
+44 2074092001
www.the-refinery.com
Opening hours .... Open 7 days
Booking .... Telephone

TOMMY GUNS
49 Charlotte Road
London EC2A 3QT, England
+44 2077392244
www.tommyguns.co.uk
Opening hours .... Closed Sunday
Booking .... Online and telephone

UNITED STATES OF AMERICA

BAXTER FINLEY
515 North La Cienega Boulevard
West Hollywood
Los Angeles, California 90048
+1 3106574726
www.baxterfinley.com
Opening hours .... Closed Monday
Booking .... Telephone

SWEENEY TODD'S BARBER SHOP
4639 Hollywood Boulevard, Los Feliz
Los Angeles, California 90027
+1 3236679690
www.sweeneytoddsbarbershopla.com
Opening hours .... Open 7 days
Booking .... Telephone

FELLOW BARBER
696 Valencia Street, Mission District
San Francisco, California 94110
+1 4153440443
www.fellowbarber.com
Opening hours .... Open 7 days
Booking .... Online

PEOPLE'S BARBER & SHOP
1259 Polk Street, Nob Hill
San Francisco, California 94109
+1 4152924099
www.peoplesbarber-sf.com
Opening hours .... Open 7 days
Booking .... Online and walk in

PUBLIC BARBER SHOP
1528 Grant Avenue, North Beach
San Francisco, California 94133
+1 4153620040
www.publicbarbersalon.com
Opening hours .... Open 7 days
Booking .... Online and telephone

PROFESSIONAL BARBERSHOP
97 Pratt Street
Hartford, Connecticut 06103
+1 8602473795
www.professionalbarbershop.com
Opening hours .... Closed Sunday
Booking .... Telephone and walk in

JUNIOR & HATTER
Wynwood Building
2750 North West 3rd Avenue
Miami, Florida 33127
+1 3055718361
www.juniorandhatter.com
Opening hours .... Closed Sunday
Booking .... Telephone

SLOANE SQUARE BARBERS
& SHOPPE
1322 Alton Road
Miami Beach, Florida 33139
+1 3056730877
www.sloanesq.com
Opening hours .... Closed Sunday
Booking .... Telephone and email

THE SHAVE BARBER SHOP
630 North Highland Avenue
Atlanta, Georgia 30306
+1 4045650730
www.theshavebarber.com
Opening hours .... Closed Monday
Booking .... No bookings

MOJO BARBERSHOP
1157 Bethel Street
Honolulu, Hawaii 96813
+1 8089278017
www.mojobarbershop.com
Opening hours .... Closed Sunday
Booking .... Telephone

RED'S CLASSIC BARBER SHOP CO.
22 East Washington Street
Indianapolis, Indiana 46204
+1 3176367337
www.redsclassicbarbershop.com

Opening hours .... Open 7 days
Booking .... Online and telephone

AIDAN GILL FOR MEN
2026 Magazine Street
New Orleans, Louisiana 70130
+1 5045879090
www.aidangillformen.com
Opening hours .... Open 7 days
Booking .... Telephone

BARBERSHOP LOUNGE
245 Newbury Street
Boston, Massachusetts 02116
+1 6174500021
www.barbershoplounge.com
Opening hours .. Closed Monday & Sunday
Booking .... Telephone

BLIND BARBER
339 East 10th Street
Manhattan, New York 10009
+1 2122282123
www.blindbarber.com
Opening hours .... Open 7 days
Booking .... Online

CLEMENTE & POLO
Ralph Lauren Mansion
650 Madison Avenue
Manhattan, New York 10022
+1 2126446189
Opening hours .... By request
Booking .... By referral only

FELLOW BARBER
101 North 8th Street
Brooklyn, New York 11249
+1 7185224959
www.fellowbarber.com
Opening hours .... Open 7 days
Booking .... Online

FREEMANS SPORTING CLUB BARBER
8 Rivington Street
Manhattan, New York 10002
+1 2122561309

www.freemanssportingclub.com
Opening hours .... Open 7 days
Booking .... Online

HARRY'S CORNER SHOP
64 MacDougal Street
Manhattan, New York 10012
+1 6469645193
www.harrys.com/cornershop
Opening hours .... Open 7 days
Booking .... Online

PERSONS OF INTEREST
82–84 Havemeyer Street
Brooklyn, New York 11211
+1 7182189100
www.personsofinterestbklyn.com
Opening hours .... Open 7 days
Booking .... Telephone and email

RUDY'S BARBERSHOP
Ace Hotel
14 West 29th Street
Manhattan, New York 10001
+1 2125327200
www.rudysbarbershop.com
Opening hours .... Open 7 days
Booking .... Online

OLD FAMILIAR BARBERSHOP
116 Parsons Avenue
Columbus, Ohio 43215
+1 6142231325
www.oldfamiliarbarbershop.com
Opening hours .... Closed Wednesday
Booking .... Telephone

THE MODERN MAN
4538 Southeast Hawthorne Boulevard
Portland, Oregon 97215
+1 5038583219
Opening hours .... Open 7 days
Booking .... Telephone

BIRD'S BARBERSHOP
905 East 41st Street
Austin, Texas 78751
+1 5124928400
www.birdsbarbershop.com
Opening hours .... Open 7 days
Booking .... Telephone and walk in

THE GENT'S PLACE
10720 Preston Road
Dallas, Texas 75230
+1 2143290400
www.thegentsplace.com
Opening hours .... Open 7 days
Booking .... Online and telephone

RUDY'S BARBERSHOP
614 East Pine Street
Seattle, Washington 98122
+1 2063293008
www.rudysbarbershop.com
Opening hours .... Open 7 days
Booking .... Online

BARBER OF HELL'S BOTTOM
818 Rhode Island Avenue N.W.
Washington DC 20001
+1 2023320200
www.barberofhellsbottom.com
Opening hours .... Closed Sunday
Booking .... Telephone

CREDITS

Phaidon Press Limited
Regent's Wharf
All Saints Street
London N1 9PA

Phaidon Press Inc.
65 Bleecker Street
New York, NY 10012

www.phaidon.com

First published in English 2016
© 2016 Phaidon Press Limited

ISBN 978 0 7148 7104 2

Original title: *Barber Couture* © 2014 24 ORE Cultura Srl

This edition published by Phaidon Press Limited under license from 24 ORE Cultura Srl
© 2014 24 ORE Cultura Srl

Original Italian edition edited by Giulia Pivetta with illustrations by Matteo Guarnaccia

Commissioning Editor: Emilia Terragni
Project Editor: Joe Pickard
Production Controller: Steven Bryant
Designed by Hans Stofregen
Editorial assistance: Maya Birke von Graevenitz
Copyeditor: Tamsin Perrett

Printed in China